Krzysztof Dziewanowski
Radosław Drozd

Cogito ergo sum

Krzysztof Dziewanowski
Radosław Drozd

Cogito ergo sum

LAP LAMBERT Academic Publishing

Imprint

Cover image: www.ingimage.com

Publisher:
LAP LAMBERT Academic Publishing
is a trademark of
International Book Market Service Ltd., member of OmniScriptum Publishing Group
17 Meldrum Street, Beau Bassin 71504, Mauritius

Printed at: see last page
ISBN: 978-613-9-86007-4

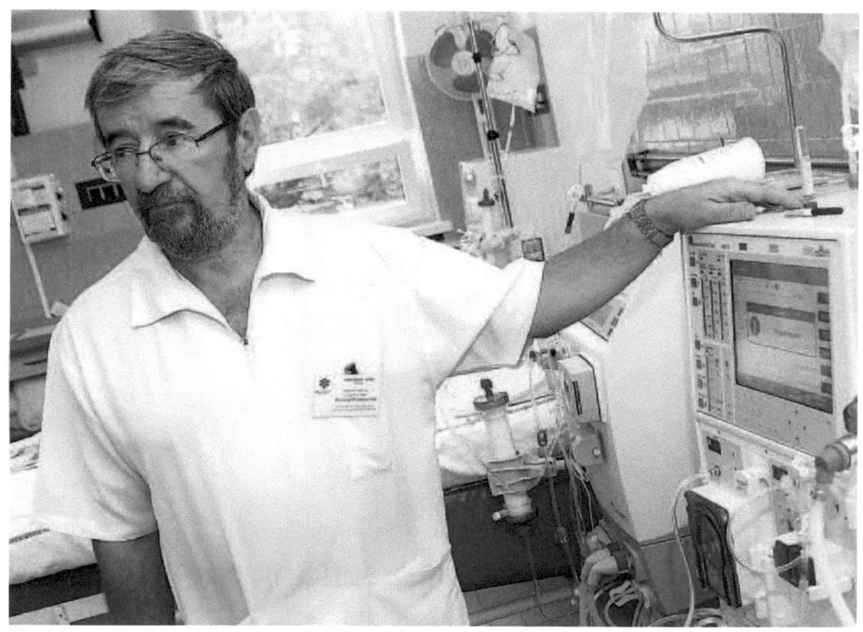

US Professor Dr. med. Krzysztof Dziewanowski born 1946 in Cracow. Medical studies completed in the Pomeranian Medical University in Szczecin (Poland) in 1970, a specialist in internal medicine, nephrology and clinical transplantation. Longtime head of the Centre for Nefrological Transplantation Regional Hospital in Szczecin and researcher at the University of Szczecin, the author of about 100 publications and several patents and inventions.

Dr. med . Radosław Drozd is a long-term nephrologist and clinical transplantologist. For over a dozen years he has been cooperating clinically and scientifically with Professor Krzysztof Dziewanowski. He is the author and co-author of many reports and scientific presentations.

Krzysztof Dziewanowski, Radosław Drozd

Cogito ergo sum

Some ideas of practicing nephrologists

Contents

The authors would like to thank all those who helped and supported the above book. Thank you especially:

- prof. inż. Henrykowi Dziewanowskiemu (posthumously)

- inż. Piotrowi Radionowi (firm Radex)

- inż. Jerzemu Dziewanowskiemu

- prof. Stanisławowi Czekalskiemu

- prof. Markowi Ostrowskiemu

- prof. Bogusławowi Machalińskiemu

- prof. Markowi Myślakowi

- dr Małgorzacie Klinke

- dr Elżbiecie i dr Andrzejowi Krzystolikom

- dr Anastasowi Skurasowi i dr Andreassis Goetzemich

Without their help, this book would be much more modest, or not be created at all.

INTRODUCTION

The last decades have been characterized by the turbulent development of many fields of science, including a significant progress in the diagnosis and treatment of patients. This was especially true in two areas of medicine: cardiology and nephrology. It is generally accepted that especially nephrology is the horse of modern medicine. Various currently used methods of renal replacement therapy: hemodialysis, peritoneal dialysis (ADO, CADO), and finally kidney transplants taken from both deceased and living donors caused that patients with renal affection may live for several decades. Currently, several million patients are treated with these methods in the world and their number is constantly growing. At the same time, more and more optimal methods and therapeutic methods are being sought to improve the comfort and survival time of these patients.

The authors of this publication have been dealing with the above problems for almost half a century. In addition, they are constantly looking for and are trying to implement their own individual ideas that can improve the diagnosis and treatment results of such patients. Some of their concepts are presented in this book. Some of them have already been presented at medical conferences or in professional literature. Nevertheless, the authors believe that wider access to their readers may be helpful in deepening this subject matter and may also increase the chance of their application in practice. They also count on discussion and invite to cooperation.

In general, the book can be divided into two main parts: plans for own diagnostic and therapeutic concepts such as: plasma dialysis, use of constant magnetic field during hemodialysis to reduce heparinization, dynamic assessment of blood clotting times during dialysis, bladder dialysis, and external voltage measurements internal to transplanted kidneys. The second part deals with such practical therapeutic issues as: treatment of patients with chronic renal failure and secondary severe hyperparathyroidism, use or even discontinuation of suppression after renal transplantation when donors are identical twins, the need to monitor blood levels after transplantation of immunosuppressive drugs (especially mycophenolate mofetil), and also based on their own good transplantation results, an attempt to analyze the factors that may decide about the optimization of the improvement of the treatment results of these patients.

Plasma dialysis –what it is?

INTRODUCTION

Plasma dialysis, which involves separation of blood cells from the plasma before the dialyzer, allowing only for the passage of plasma through the dialyzer canal. The aim of this study was to suggest novel model of high efficacy plasma dialysis as hemodialysis alternative. Electron microscopy imaging of the capillary lumens following an investigation plasma dialysis and hemodialysis were performed. Full blood clearance index was calculated, basing on the percent reduction of creatinine level before and after the dialysis both for the typical hemodialysis and plasma dialysis. Visualization of the plasma dialysis procedure indication decrease in the number of attached blood cells of compared to the hemodialysis. Creatinine clearance index ranged 79-86% for the hemodialysis and decreased over time during the procedure, while for plasma dialysis ranged from 94 to 95%. Also, no decreasing trend in procedure efficacy over time was found. Based on the experimental data two models for dialyzers were designed: rotary dialyzer and dialyzer with double capillary walls. Plasma dialysis may allow for the improved plasma clearance with estimated about 20% higher efficacy compared to the hemodialysis based systems, be useful in the setting of relatively low blood flow (for example 100-150 ml/min) and may reduce duration and frequency of dialysis procedures.

Currently it is clear that adequate degree of dialysis of patients with chronic renal failure not only prolongs their survival, but also results in reduction of atherosclerosis progression and improves their immunity against infections or malignancies, eventually resulting in reduction of treatment costs. Therapy of such patients is multifactorial. Essentially it can be divided into medical treatment (maintenance and forcing residual urine output, using an optimal diet and fluid supply, treating an underlying disease, controlling potential infection foci, treating abnormalities of erythropoiesis, lipid metabolism, calcium-phosphate) and procedural treatment (renal replacement therapy). Improved degree of dialysis in these patients during repeated hemodialysis can be achieved by, among others: increased duration and frequency of dialysis procedures, increased blood flow through the blood channel in the dialyzer to a maximum value, increased flow of the dialyzing fluid, use of dialyzers with large exchange areas, dialysis through two-needle access, alternating hemodialysis and hemodiafiltration procedures.

However, all these methods are not universally effective, in particular in patients with poor vascular access (with low efficiency) or those who poorly tolerate increased dialysis duration or frequency. In such cases the treatment of choice may involve plasma dialysis as suggested in this study. Plasma dialysis is based on the principle of removing the plasma and passing through the extracorporeal medical device for the purpose of separation of the cellular components from the blood. After separation, cellular components are re-infused to the system. It is also effective in removal of soluble immune complexes, modulate humoral response and decrease the titers of the autoantibodies, inflammatory modulators providing beneficial effect on the endothelial function and immune regulation. Its most common uses so far have included anti-GBM nephritis, cryoglobulinemia, or hemolytic-uremic syndrome, where removal of the circulating toxic factors is essential.

MATERIALS AND METHODES.

Here, we wish to present the concept of solution based on an assumption that diffusion of toxic compounds from the full blood to the dialyzing fluid may be hindered by the presence of blood cells that adhere to pores in the dialyzing membrane and impair the above mentioned process (Fig. 1). The aim of this study is to propose the new model of plasma dialysis and compare its efficacy to the conventional hemodialysis procedure.

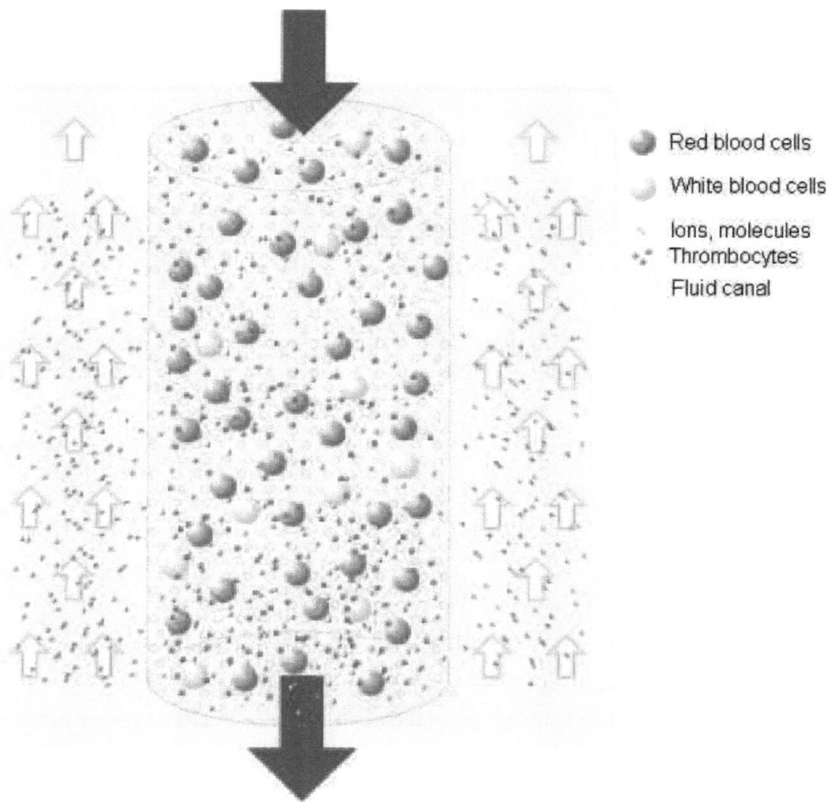

Fig. 1. Model of blood flow in the dialyzer capillary.

We have created the concept model of plasma dialysis, involving separation blood cells from the plasma before the dialyzer, allowing only for the passage of plasma through the dialyzer canal. After the filtration step, plasma is returned to be combined with previously separated blood cells before its re-infusion to the patient body (Fig. 2). For the dialyses and hemodialysis the Fresenius 4008 S device was used.

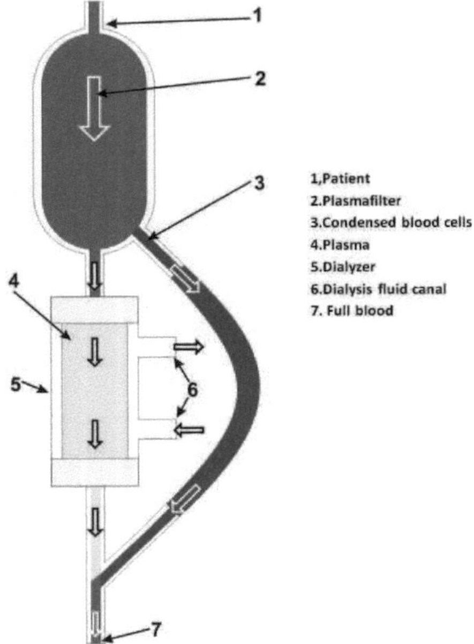

Fig. 2. Schematic presentation of the presented plasma dialysis.

Firstly, based on these assumptions, comparison of images of internal capillary walls obtain using an electron microscope after typical hemodialysis were performed. This stage of the study included images of the dialyzer capillary after passage of the peritoneal cavity trans due from of female patient with uncontrolled liver cirrhosis who participates in a program of repeated hemodialysis. All images were obtained under the same flow conditions and using the capillary and hemodialyzer model. Obtained images are presented on figures 3-6, demonstrating internal lumens of dialyzing capillaries under various magnifications, following a conventional hemodialysis.

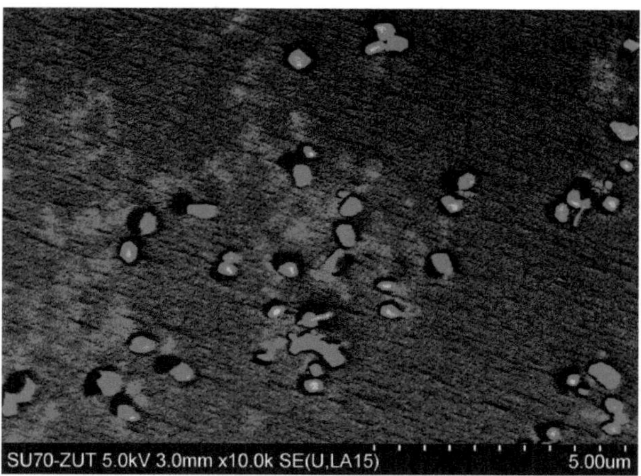

Fig. 3. Light capillary dialyzer after hemodialysis (electron microscope 5 000).

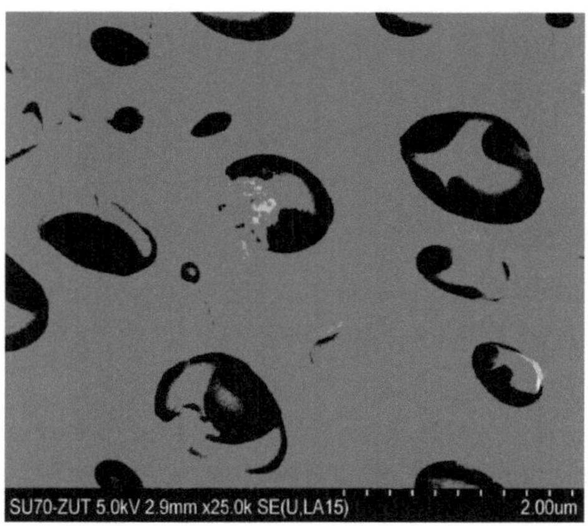

Fig. 4. Light capillary dialyzer after hemodialysis (electron microscope 50 000x).

Secondly, imaging of the capillary lumens following an investigation plasma dialysis, were performed. For this purpose, standard imaging procedure with the scanning electron microscope Zeiss LEO was used. Comparison of capillary lumens from an electron microscope (magnification 50 000x) after a typical hemodialysis and after a plasma dialysis procedure is also presented and indicates decrease in the number of attached blood cells.

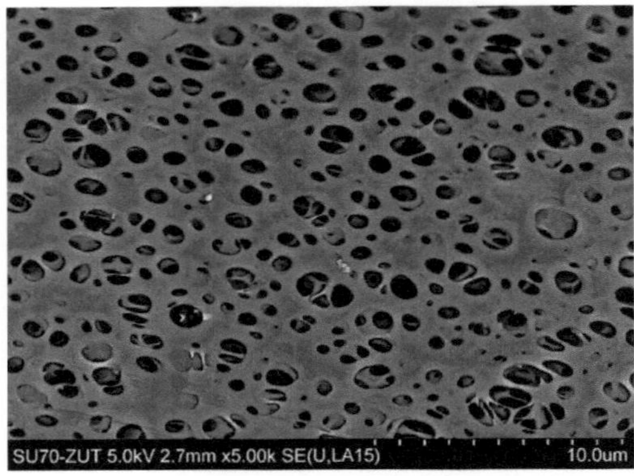

Fig. 5. Light capillary dialyzer after plasma dialysis (electron microscope 20000x).

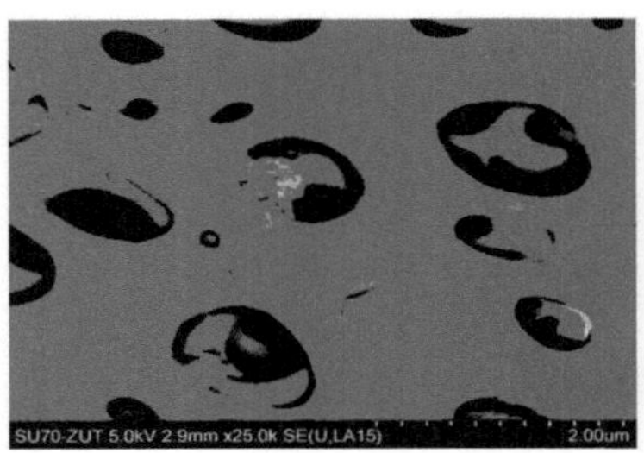
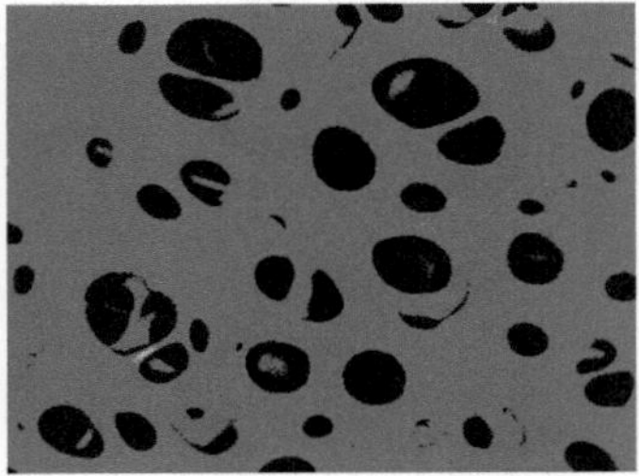

Fig. 6. Light capillary dialyzer after hemodialysis (electron microscope 50 000x) and light capillary dialyzer after plasma dialysis (electron microscope 30 000x).

Subsequently a full blood clearance index was calculated, basing on the percent reduction of creatinine level before and after the dialysis both for the typical hemodialysis and an investigation plasma dialysis (Fig. 7-8).

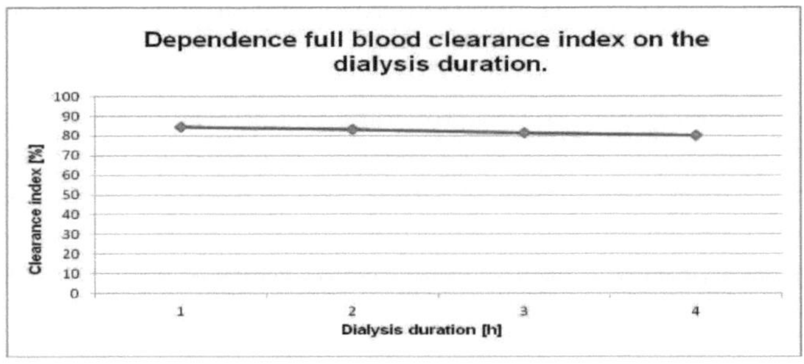

Fig. 7. Association between creatinine clearance index and time hemodialysis.

This index ranged 79-86% for the full blood and decreased over time during procedure, while was higher for plasma dialysis and ranged from 94-95%; furthermore, no trend towards its reduction during the procedure was found.

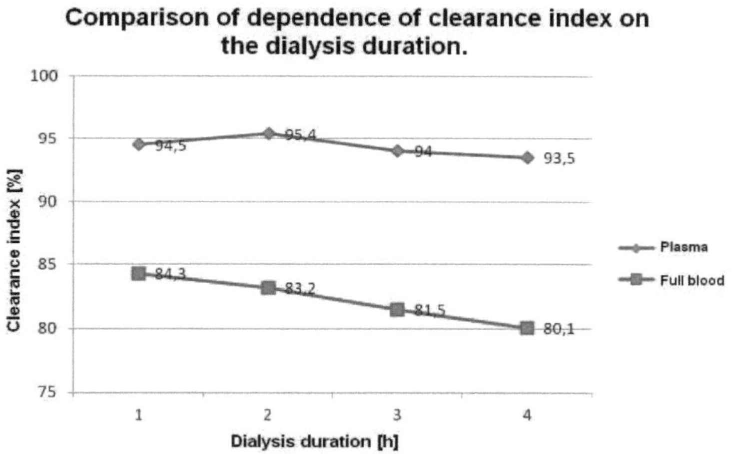

Fig. 8. Comparison of clearance index efficacy over time for hemodialysis and plasma dialysis.

Based on these observations we may predict that suggested method of blood clearance may be more effective if compared to the conventional hemodialysis. In theory, one could perform the above mentioned plasma dialysis procedure using a parallel connection of a typical plasma filter and a dialyzer. However, such system would require withdrawal of a large amount of blood from the patients circulation (which may not always prove beneficial), while commercially available plasma filters provide relatively small amounts of separated plasma (up to approximately 50 ml/min), which would be insufficient.

Taking into consideration these practical aspects, we wish to suggest the concept for construction of a new dialyzer type. This dialyzer would simultaneously perform a process of separation of plasma and blood cells and perform the dialysis. Here we present two variants of such solution: rotary dialyzer (Fig. 9) and dialyzer with double capillary walls (Fig. 10).

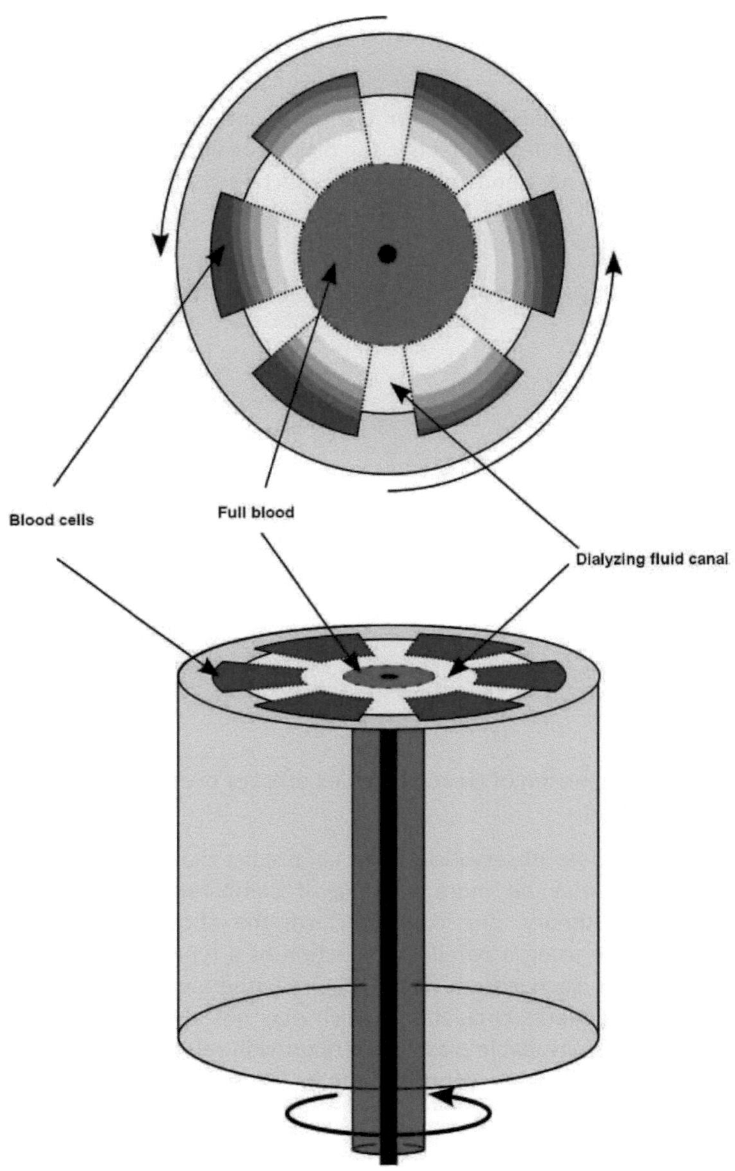

Fig. 9. Rotary dialyzer.

Such dialyzer would rotate during the procedure, resulting in accumulation of blood cells on its walls, while the plasma would remain in the central part and would be cleared through contact with flowing dialyzing fluid. Possible problems with manufacturing of such dialyzer include constructional problems and need to maintain leak-proof system both in the blood canal and fluid canal.

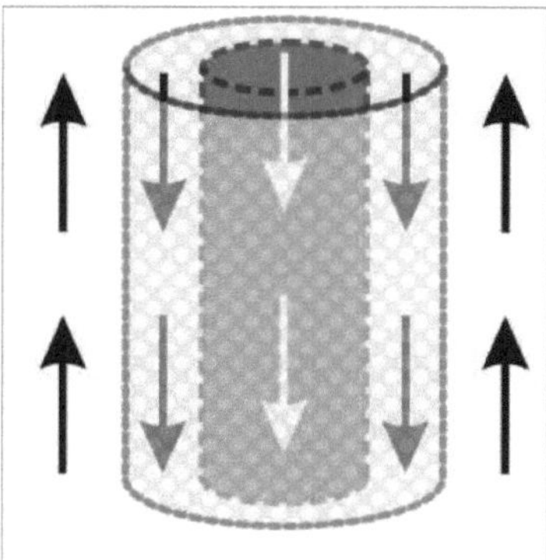

Fig. 10. Dialyzer with double capillary walls.

With this approach, full blood would flow through an inner capillary. Its walls would possess pores (approximately 3000 000 kDa in diameter) allowing the fluid part of the blood, plasma, to be evacuated outside this component. Plasma flowing through this space would contact a dialyzing fluid through typical dialyzing membrane (pores approximately 15 000 D in diameter) and would be cleared conventionally. We believe that such construction of a plasma dialyzer could be optimal.

This study presents a concept model for the plasma dialysis with the separation of the cellular blood components prior to the entry into the dialysis capillary. Benefits of this systems include stable efficacy and stability in time. The system was indicated to allow for the stable creatinine clearance. Construction of such devices may result in the progress of the dialysis methods and improvement of patient care. Following the construction of such plasma dialyzers and required clinical trials these devices may contribute to the following:

Improved plasma clearance if compared to the full blood, with estimated 20% higher efficacy compared to the hemodialysis based systems, efficient dialysis of patients even with relatively low blood flow (for example 100-150 ml/min) and low blood pressure, the duration and frequency of dialysis procedures could be notably reduced in selected patients. In the available literature we did not find the proposed similar solutions in terms of improving the efficiency of hemodialysis, which may indicate that it is our individual project. Undoubtedly, this concept requires further study, debate and attempts to design a new prototype capillary dialyzer. Initial assumptions of our project were presented in the polish medical magazines.

Conclusions: Presented dialysis methodology is a concept for the improvement of dialysis. Its key features include better plasma clearance and higher efficacy compared to hemodialysis as well as possibility to use in the setting of the decreased blood flow and pressure.

References:

1. Orlandi G.C.,Margaria R.: Evaluation of the efficiency of a new hollow fiber plasmapheresis filter. Int.J. Artif. Organs. 1983;(supl.1):103-106.

2. Kale-Pradhan PB., Woo MH.: A review of the effects of plasmapheresis on drug clearance. Pharmacotherapy 1997,17,684.

3. Kaplan AA.: General principles of therapeutic plasma exchange. Semin.Dial. 1995,8,294.

4. Kaplan AA.: Plasma exchange for non-renal indications. Semin. Dial. 1996,9, 265.

5. Tan H.K.,Hart G.: Plasma filtration. Ann.Acad.Med. Singapure 2005;34: 615-624.

6. Madore F.: Therapeutic plasma exchange in renal diseases. J.Am.Soc.Nephrol.1996,7,367.

7. Hajme N.,Machiko A.,Atsunori K. et al.: A case report of efficiency of double filtration plasmapheresis in treatment of Goodpasture,s syndrome. Ther. Apher.Dial.2009;13:373-377.

8. Madore F. : Plasmapheresis technical aspects and indications. Crit. Care Clin. 2002,18,375.

9. Mokrzycki MH., Kaplan AA.: Therapeutic Plasma Exchange: Complications and Management . Am.J.Kidney DIS. 1994,23,817.

10. Nenov D.,Metodiev K.: Combined treatment immune nephropathies with plasmapheresis and immunosuppressants. Biomater. Artif.Cells Artif.Organs 1988-1989;16:991-997.

11. Weinstein R.: Is there a scientific rationale for therapeutic plasma exchange or intravenous immune globin in the treatment of acute Guillian-Barre syndrome? J.Clin. Apheresis 1995,10,150.

12. Weinstein R.: Prevention of citrate reaction during therapeutic plasma exchange by constant infusion of calcium gluconate with return fluid. J.Clin.Apheresis. 1996,11,204.

13. Dziewanowski K.,Drozd R.: Plazmadializa jako alternatywna metoda poprawy stopnia wydializowania chorych z przewlekłą niewydolnością nerek. Forum Nefrologiczne.2013 (3):150.

1. MONITORING OF BLOOD CLOTTING DURING HEMODIALYSIS – NEED OR NECESSITY?

ABSTRACT

Contemporary "artificial kidney" has a whole set of security rules assure the efficiency and safety of the treatment. Prevention of blood clotting in bloodline, usually based on the administration of adequate doses of heparin, which amount shall be determined individually based primarily on such parameters as body weight, morphological composition of blood clotting time of assessment or part-time and activated tromboplastyn a-PTT. Typically, such a procedure is sufficient. There are however, situations where the use heparin, especially in the average doses of dangerous or even contraindicated. This applies especially to patients after fresh surgery (eg, after renal transplantation), patients with fresh bleeding into the gastrointestinal tract and central nervous system, etc. In such cases, often decide to dialysis with minimal heparinization or even dialysis without heparin. Other methods of anticoagulation, such as dialysis with heparin and protamine neutralization whether the use citrate neutralized by administration of calcium, are used with a variety of reasons, relatively rare. Currently, the marked could not have come dialysers permanently heparinized (Evodol), but they also only allow for 30% of the surgery without the use heparin. In such situations, a need for continuous monitoring of coagulation in patients during hemodialysis particularly becomes useful. The problem is even more important that the evaluation of the coagulation system during routine laboratory testing get at best, after dozen, tens minutes, during which time the conditions of blood clotting in the blood line can be dramatically changed. The above was a prerequisite for their own work and trials in this area.

Research methods.

Planned and pre-checked experimentally, using its own collection of blood from researches, the relationship between the number of drops of blood per minute (at a constant positive flow of blood flow through the line), and coagulation lime designated by Lee-White and a-PTT. We found close linear relationship of these parameters: decrease over time in the study and depletion of the added activity at the start of heparin, time a-PTT parallel decrease in the blood drops/minute as a result of increased viscosity. The statement of this relationship could be used to construct the device numbering (at constant flow rates during hemodialysis) the number of drops of blood in one minute to the relevant coagulation parameters (spectroscopic measurements, photocell, computer, monitor).

Another proposed method of measurement is due at time found their own tests and depending on the time a-PTT and called dynamic viscosity of blood. We have shown, and with time study and the depletion of heparin-added activity, and time a-PTT decreases, while the coefficient of dynamic viscosity increases considerably. There is a close linear dependence of these parameters, which increases the resistance within the blood lines, and thereby increase the pressure difference between the influence of the outflow of blood to the patient. It led to necessity that can be monitored during hemodialysis blood clotting process, not only by measuring the clotting, but also alter its viscosity. This therefore became the motivation for constructing a model of such a device (diagram included in the rest application), which would be the most important element of a differential manometer showing the change in blood pressure in the line before and after dialyzer. The increase in resistance found on the gauge would be converted to computer-coagulation parameters and displayed on the monitor (with appropriate gating, alarm possibilities, and ultimately controlled administration of heparin).

Modern artificial kidney contains a number of security and regulations ensuring the safety of patients during hemodialysis. In the available writing does not come across any project device that provides dynamic monitoring of the process of coagulation of blood during the surgery, which would be particularly important in patients treated with traditional heparization, and which recently after operating in the treatment after kidney transplantation, with active bleeding, blemish hemorrhagic etc. It is a strong motivation to our work in this area. We found experimentally that there is a close relationship between:

- number of drops of blood and clotting (in side branch blood line) at steady flow (Figure 1)

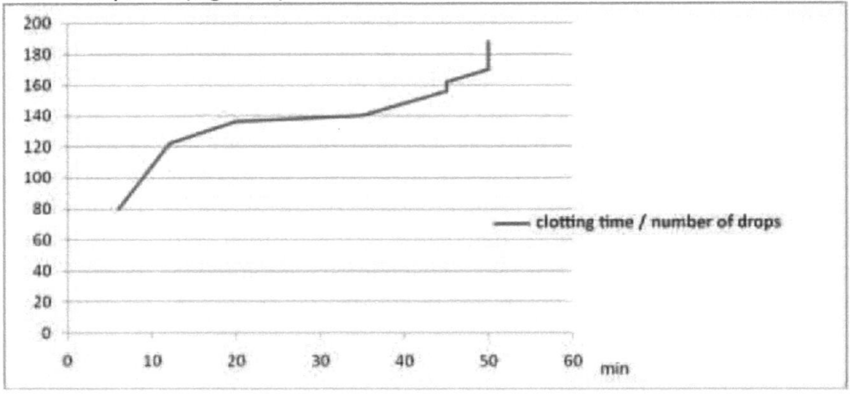

- and between and viscosity of blood (the coefficient of dynamic viscosity) and sometimes a-PTT (Figure 2)

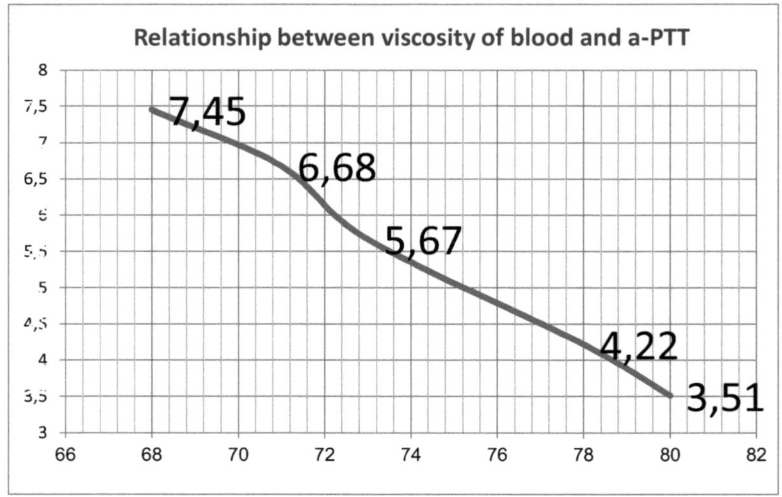

These observations have become a basis fir the concept to construct two variants of apparatus, which in the form of attachment can be used for dynamic valuation of changing during hemodialysis treatment clotting of blood.

A Variant I

A draft of such a device is shown in figure 3. In a side branch of a typical line of blood used for haemodialysis, that granted permanent low blood flow (pressure passing blood in this branch would be permanent, controlled by the valve up) installed would be counter photometric major dynamic number of drops of blood per minute. These data are then transmitted to the computer converting the amount of time a-PTT, and then displayed on a device that monitors and joined with control adequate supply prepared in advance of heparin. Of course, the device would also monitor the relevant regulating and gating the desired parameters of coagulation.

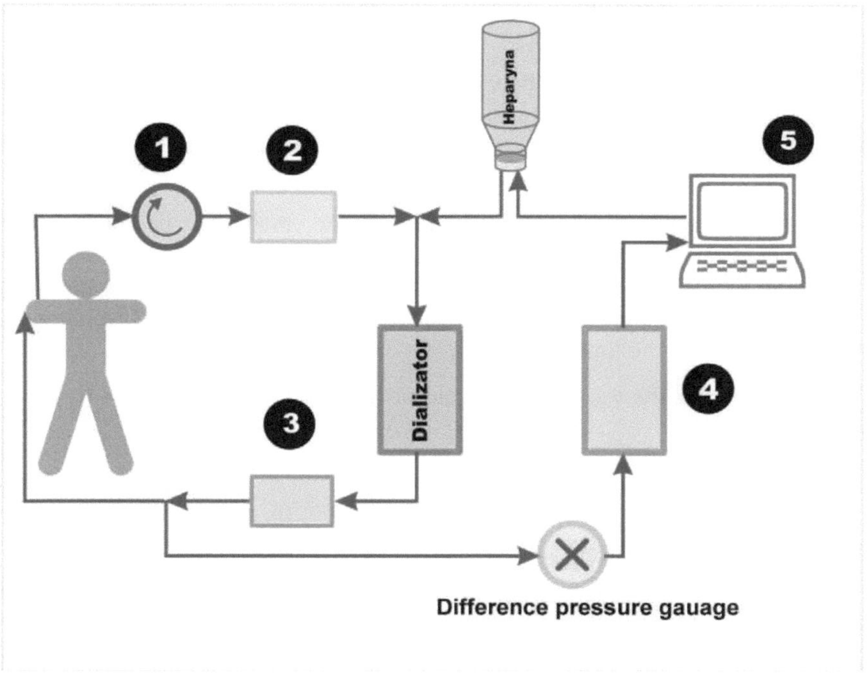

1 – pump of blood,
2,3 – vents,
4- dropper with a photocell,
5 – computer converts the measured number of drops of blood on the aPTT, specifying the dose of heparin administered.

A Variant II

In relation to any previous relationship between linear time and a viscosity of blood clotting and, in this variant will be based on indications the differential pressure gauge installed on lines of blood before and past dialyzer (Figure 3). Change the difference in pressure between the evaluate points of the line of blood, the machine will be count at an appropriate time a-PTT, which in turn would be joined with the monitoring and device control an appropriate supply of heparin.

Any design and technical difficulties that may arise in the implementation of this policy option. The complexity of the method. The need for modernization of the blood.

Concerns or slow blood flow in the side branch blood line with dropper (a significant difference in diameter tubing) no significant impact on the final result of the measurement coagulation (the need to introduce appropriate amendments).

The present method of measurement may be useful in the implementation of the final design of the instrument that is used to continuously monitor the coagulation of blood during hemodialysis (measuring the change in blood pressure before and after the dialyzer judge also alter its viscosity and thus the time a-PTT).

Monitoring the viscosity of the blood during hemodialysis

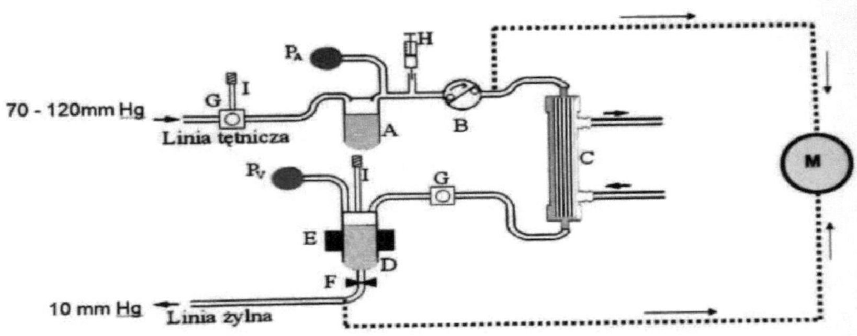

A - arterial expansion tank, B – pump of blood, C – dialyzer, D – venosus expansion tank, E - ultrasonic air detector, F - detector with clamp lock, G - ports of the window for blood, H - heparin infusion pump, I - infusion ports, M - differential pressure gauges.

The proposed device would enter the following: a redesigned line of blood, differential pressure gauge, pressure transducer for blood lines drawn dispensing appropriate dose heparin, computer converts the differential pressure on the a-PTT with monitoring devices and the control processor supply of heparin.

We hope that the construction of the two variants of the project, would allow us to choose after proper clinical trials of an optimal model, its eventual replacement, and in the long start up domestic production of the first copies of the project.

References:

1. Johansson PI: Coagulation monitoring of the bleeding traumatized patient. Curr. Opin. Anaesthesiol.: 2012, Apr.25(2), 235-41

2. Kuznik Bl., Fine IW., Kaminsky AV.: A noninvasive method of examination of the hemostatis system. Bull. Exp. Biol.Med 2011, Sep.151(5) 655-57

3. Hitosugi M., Kawato H., Nagai T I wsp.: Changes in blood viscosity with heavy and light exercise. Med.Sci.Law. 2004, Jul,44(3), 197-200

4. Puckett LG., Barrett G., Kouzoudis D. i wsp.: Monitoring blood coagulation with magnetoelastic sensors. Biosens Bioelectron. 2003, May, 18(5-6), 675-81

5. Canaud B., Bragg-Gresham J.L, Marshall M.R I wsp.: Patient receiving hemodiafiltration versus hemodialysis. European results from the DOPPS, Kidney Int. 2006, 69, 2087-93

6. Finkel K.W., Foringer J.R.: Safety of regional citrate anticoagulation for continuous sustained low efficacy dialysis in critically ill patients. Ren.Fail.2005,27,541-45

7. Ouseph R., Ward R.A Anticoagulation for intermittent hemodialysis. Semin. Dial. 2000, 13,181-87

8. Caruana R.J.: Heparin-free dialysis: comparative data and results in high-risk patients. Kidney Int. 1987, 31, 1351-56

9. Bagling T., Barrowcliffe T.W., Cohen A .: Guidelines on the use and monitoring of heparin. Br.J.Hem. 2006, 133,19-34

Influence of Static Magnetic Field on Blood Coagulation in Patients Treated with Hemodialysis.

Magnetic energy is one of the most important factors influencing life on Earth. Most of biological processes in the human body are dependent on electromagnetic forces generated by magnetic field. In the available literature there are few reports about the influence of magnetic field on the process of blood coagulation in humans.

The aim of our study was to evaluate the impact of static magnetic field (set of Multimag magnets) on the process of blood clotting time measured with APTT (partial thromboplastin time) in patients treated with hemodialysis. Approximately 350-400 ml of blood was drawn from patients with renal transplant and erythrocytosis. Small amount of heparin was added to this blood. Then the resulting volume was divided into two equal parts. Two identical dialyzers and blood lines were filled with this blood. Identical flow of blood was forced through both sets, while one of those sets was equipped with Multimag magnet (0, 1 Tesla). Samples of blood were collected from both lines and a PTT was assessed in each of them. There was significant shortening of a PTT time (average about 30%) in sets without magnets as compared to the lines carrying Multimag. Tests carried out have shown that the magnetic field produced by the magnet system (Multimag) planted on a typical blood line used in hemodialyzed patients, significantly prolonged blood clotting time evaluated by a PTT and thus prolonged the ability to continue treatment as compared with sets without magnets.

The aim of our study was to evaluate influence of static magnetic field of 0.1 Tesla magnitude produced by a set of Multimag magnets (U.S. Patent 6, 143, 0450) on blood clotting in the device used for hemodialysis used in patients with renal failure.

In 10 patients with kidney transplants and erythrocytosis, at the time of regular follow-up outpatient visits, after controlling complete blood counts and establishing clinical

indication for phlebotomy, 350-400 ml of blood was collected, to which 100 ml of 0.9% NaCl and 0.5 mg of heparin were added. The resulting solution was divided into two equal parts, then two identical typical bloodlines with common polynephronic capillary dialyzers (Nipro -Elisio 170M with 1.7 square meter exchange area) were filled with the solution. Both sets were then connected to two identical dialyzers, forcing identical blood flow at the rate of 100ml/min with the use of pumps. One blood line was permanently equipped (before dialyzer) with Multimag magnet (0.1 Tesla). Blood samples were collected from both lines simultaneously every 2-3 hours and a-PTT (sec.) was measured. (Fig. 1, 2).

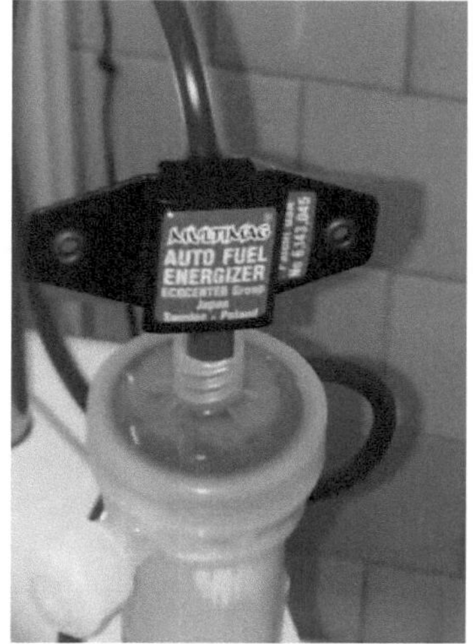

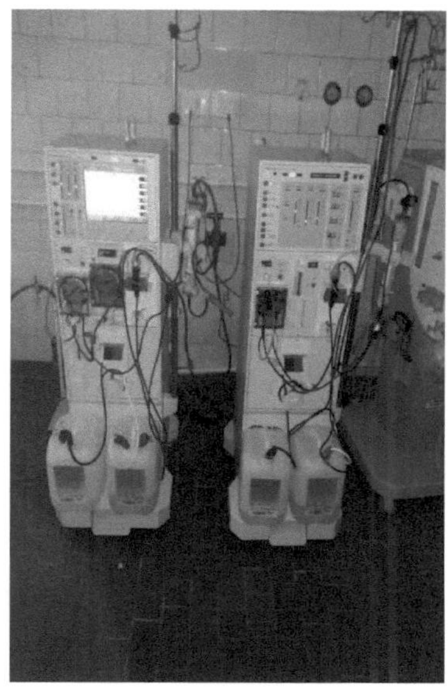

Figure 1. Multimag blood line. **Figure 2.** Test and control.

At the beginning of our measurements we have found that after over a dozen of hours coagulation of blood took place in the line of the kidney dialyzer without the magnet, while in the line with Multimag magnet this did not occur or it happened with a considerable delay. Further observations demonstrated a significant decrease in a-PTT time (on the average about 30%) in lines without the magnets in comparison to lines with Multimags, and there was a significant correlation between the two sets of results (0.973) Fig. 3.

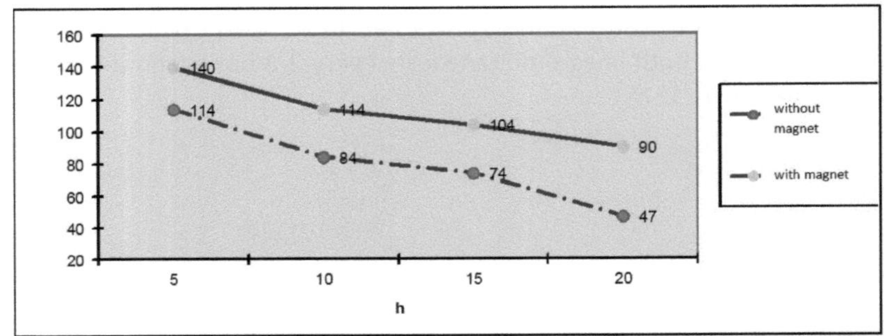

Figure 3. Comparison of a-PTT with and without magnetization.

Table 1. Without Mg (time a-PTT – sec.).

Time (h)											Average	SD
5	140	136	144	144	139	135	142	143	137	140	140	3, 4641016
10	114	110	118	112	114	115	108	121	114	114	114	3, 9051248
15	104	100	109	108	106	99	98	107	105	104	104	4, 0620192
20	90	88	86	94	92	90	97	84	89	90	90	3, 968627

Table 2. With Mg (time a-PTT – sec.).

Time (h)											Average	SD
5	113	110	116	119	110	115	114	115	114	114	114	2, 828427
10	86	88	89	82	82	80	84	84	81	84	84	3, 122499
15	74	75	74	72	70	79	74	75	73	74	74	2, 44949
20	47	48	49	46	45	47	43	49	49	47	47	2, 061553

With Mg/ Out Mg p = 0, 003

There was a significant shortening of APTT time (average about 30%) in sets without magnets as compared to the lines carrying Multimag. Tests carried out have shown that the magnetic field produced by the magnet system (Multimag) planted on a typical blood line used in hemodialyzed patients, significantly prolonged blood clotting time evaluated by APTT and thus prolonged the ability to continue treatment as compared with sets without magnets.

"Magnetic energy is the elementary energy which determines life on Earth, "these words of Nobel prize winner Werner Hesenberg help us to realize the importance of this issue. Proper human magnetic field (biofield) is produced by biochemical processes occurring in our body and by the action of Earth's magnetic field whose magnitude is estimated at 0.1-1.0 miliTesla

(1-10 Gauss). Absence or diminishing of this natural magnetic field exerts a number of adverse effects on the human body. This is confirmed by examinations of astronauts - orbital station workers, who stay a long time outside the natural magnetic field of the Earth. Attempts to fix this issue are done by equipping their spacesuits with magnets. It is widely believed that the north pole of the Earth (negative) is more beneficial for human organisms than the south pole (positive). In the last two centuries, there was a significant weakening of Earth's magnetic field (possibly through influence of solar activity). According to some authors this explains increased predisposition to certain diseases.

Another factor disrupting our biofield is the "electromagnetic smog" produced by relay stations, radio and television waves, high voltage lines, computers, laptops, cell phones, etc. Clinical signs of disruption of our biofield are numerous and often unspecific: headache, increased fatigue, impaired concentration (Alzheimer's disease?), drowsiness or sleep disorders, neuroses, impaired libido, decreased immunity (infectious diseases), increased predisposition to cancer (leukemia in children), etc.

Beneficial effect of magnets was already appreciated by our ancestors. Magnets were considered as means of prolonging life in ancient Egypt. In China they were described as a stone of health, and in ancient Greece, they were called "stone of life". Paracelsus advocated wearing magnets due to their beneficial effects on the psyche and to aid in difficulty falling asleep. In the nineteenth century, James Clerk Maxwell demonstrated that any change in the electric field induces a change in the magnetic field and that any change in the magnetic field induces a change in the vortex electric field. He also established the first modern recommendations in magnetic field therapy. Principles of operation of the fixed and alternating magnetic field are used widely today also outside medicine (eg. fuel economy in automobile engines, linear flow of oil in pipelines - to reduce its viscosity, in initial acceleration of rockets, torpedoes, etc.).

Modern medical science has allowed to establish that physiological human biofield, among others, influences the correct polarity of cells of the body (action of the natrium-potassium pump producing a potential difference between cell membrane and cytoplasm at about 100mV), as well as physiological function of the cardiac conductive system, stimulation and inhibition in the central nervous system, intellectual processes, conduction of electrical impulses in the peripheral nervous system, etc.

Restoring or improving proper biofield is extensively used by present-day physical therapy particularly by its branches such as magnetic stimulation and magnetic therapy. Different devices (magnetic bracelets, magnetrons, Polish device "Viofor", etc.) are used for this purpose.

Both static (predominantly in the East) and alternate (predominantly in the West) magnetic field are used. It is generally accepted (according to the WHO) that treatment with these devices with magnitude prescribed for medical purposes, is safe, and its effectiveness in the treatment of, for instance, chronic pain, reaches 80%. Beneficial effect of this therapy in wound healing, treatment of injuries, fractures, as well as in neurotic or depressive conditions is emphasized.

In the available literature there are few reports about the influence of magnetic field on blood coagulation in patients.

Czajka E., et al in their work examined the influence of low frequency magnetic field used in magnetic therapy on selected parameters of coagulation in animals demonstrating significant increase in prothrombin time in the studied group of rats. Observations from the Institute of Technology in Osaka Prefecture (Japan) demonstrated that static magnetic field produced by Trion 2 magnetic bracelets used by a group of patients caused dilation of blood vessels, increased blood oxygenation, decreased adhesion and aggregation of platelets as well as reduced blood clotting.

In the available literature we did not find reports about effects of static magnetic field on blood clotting in dialyzed patients.

Reported results seem to be interesting because using our preliminary observations and after future development of the above presented idea with adjustment of used magnetic field we can be theoretically expect:

- smaller average consumption of heparin during typical hemodialysis
- a more efficient process of dialyzer reutilization,
- theoretical possibility (through anticoagulant action) to obtain a longer functioning time of dialysis catheters and fistulas,
- finally (which of course would require further research and clinical observations), beneficial effect of this method can be expected in inhibition of progression of atherosclerosis in patients, particularly with chronic renal failure treated with hemodialysis.

In summary, we conclude that use of the static magnetic field generated by the Multimag system used with typical blood lines in hemodialyzed patients significantly reduces blood coagulation evaluated with a-PTT and thereby prolongs the ability to continue treatment as compared with a magnet-free set.

References:

1. Basford J.R.: A historical perspective of the popular use of electric and magnetic therapy. Arch.Phys.Med.Rehabil. 2001,82(1), 1261-69.

2. Bąk L., Należyty-Kozak H., Dziewanowski K.: Zastosowanie magnetoterapii u chorych z pnn leczonych hemodializami. Probl.Lek.(Supl.)2004 .

3. Borowicz A.M., Kuncewicz E., Samborski W. et al.: The influence of magnetotherapy on pain symptoms In patients with chronic lower back pain. Med.Rodzinna 2008,1,2-5.

4. Czajka E., Kowacka: The influence of low magnetic field used in magnetotherapy on chosen parameters of blood clotting in experimental animals. Fizykoterapia 2004, 12,4,12-18.

5. Dąbrowski M.P., Stankiewicz W., Witkowski W.: Clinical immunological effects of magnetostymulations in children with recurrent infections of respiratory tracts. Przegl. Elektrotechniczny 2008,2,155-156.

6. Długosz T., Duziński K.: Electromagnetic environment in animal world. Ekologia i Technika 2012,2,125-130.

7. Gorczyńska E.: The effect of magnetic fields on platelets, blood coagulation and fibrinolisis in guine pigs. J.Hyg.Epidemil.Microbiol.Immunol. 1983,15 (6),459-68.

8. Kazimierska E.: Wpływ pól elektromagnetycznych na układ krzepnięcia i fibrynolizy u ludzi. Pol.Mer.Lek. 2001,55,9-11.

9. Loughran S., Mickenze R., Jackson M. et al.: Individual differences in the effects of mobile phone exposure on human sleep. Bioelectromagnetics. 2012,33, 86-91.

10. Marcinkowska-Gapińska A., Kowal P.: Próba wpływu magnetostymulacji na obraz termograficzny kończyn górnych. Neuroskop.2009,11,37-40.

11. Pasek J., Mucha R., Siroń A.: Magnetostymulacja – nowoczesna metoda terapii w medycynie i rehabilitacji. Fizykoterapia Polska. 2008,1(4),8,1-10.

12. Sieroń A., Hese R.,Sobis J.: Therapeutic efficacy of variable magnetic field with low induction value in patients with depression syndroms. IV International Congress of the European. Bioelectromagnetics Association 2003,13-15 XI. Budapest, Hungry

13. Stankiewicz W., Szymański P., Dąbrowski M.P et al.: Immunocorrective effects of magnetotherapy administered in patients with terminal injury. Przegl. Elektrotechniczny. 2009,12,49-50.

14. Sokolska G., Smigielski S.: Efekty biologiczne pól radio I mikrofalowych w badaniach doświadczalnych. Materiały Konferencyjne Pol. Tow. Radiol Zakopane.18-22 X.1993.

Automatic Dialysis of Urine Bladder – Fiction or Reality?

Nowadays we have three methods of kidney replacement therapy: hemodialysis (also hemofiltration and hemodiafiltration), peritoneal dialysis (CAPD and CCPD) and kidney transplantation (including living and deceased donor transplants). Every method has its advantages and disadvantages. We know that the best option of kidney replacement therapy is kidney transplantation. The limitation of this treatment is shortage of organs for donation, also there is a problem of many side effects of immunosuppressive drugs, like infections, cancer, diabetes, hypertension et al. Hemodialysis remains the most common therapy for people with end stage renal disease. Disadvantages of this method are problems with vascular access, catheter released infections and other. There are also many problems with the second method of dialysis treatment, peritoneal dialysis, including exit-site infections, peritonitis, peritoneal sclerosis et al. Every year we can see the progress in this kind of treatment, but there is still many problems to resolve. First of all, the peritoneal cavity is not physiologically adjusted to this kind of treatment. That's why we decided to coming up with a proposal of dialyze a urine bladder to decrease uremic toxemia in patients with end stage renal disease. The urine bladder is an integral part of urinary tract. It's capacity ranges from 250-500 ml, but it can be raised to 1000-1500 ml and even to 3000-4000 ml. The thickness of its wall is about 1 cm, but it can be diminished to 0,2 cm if the bladder is full. The bladder wall has three layers: epithelium, media and external membrane. Vascularity of the bladder is rich.

Project characterization:

The idea is to introduce dialysis solution to the urine bladder and exchange it like during peritoneal dialysis, for example with cycler. The exchange volume would depend on bladder capacity and can be limited with pain resistance. The frequency rate could be bigger than during CCPD. Dialysis solution could be introduced to the bladder using Foley's catheter. To improve vasculisation of the bladder we could use drugs, for example minoxidil.

We hope that automatic dialysis of the urine bladder can be an interesting option of the renal replacement therapy. It could be a substitute of other methods of treatment (for example in patients with low catabolism or with maintained residual renal function) or can complement and reinforce classical dialysis. Of course, many further trials using animals and then clinical trials are needed to prove efficacy and tolerability of this kind of treatment.

Internal and external pressure of transplanted kidney – on of the underestimated methods of diagnosis of renal graft.

Introduction

Hardness, tensity (tonus) of transplanted kidney can change in the course of various pathologic conditions. Manual examination (with palpation) which is most frequently used to evaluate this transplanted organ is not objective. First attempts of objective evaluation were described in medical literature in 1980s. They consisted of evaluation of intrarenal pressure by puncturing the kidney, connecting iv drip line, and measurement of pressure in centimeters of water column. Authors examined then a group of subjects revealing significant differences in mean measurements especially in patients with acute rejection process compared to the control group. However, use of this method was not continued because of its invasiveness. Our own diagnostic method, described here by authors is measurement of external kidney pressure (tonus). Two types of devices (tonometers) are described, as well as a future project of tonometer functioning on the basis of electronically measured differences in values of forces used above the graft and above the symmetrical part of the abdomen causing identical deflection of abdominal wall. 32 patients (including control group) were examined with such method. Statistically significant differences were revealed this way between patients with acute graft rejection and chronic graft nephropathy compared to the control group. Authors believe that this here described method can be a valuable supplement to other currently used noninvasive means of renal graft evaluation including ultrasonography, doppler and elastography examinations.

Transplanted kidney has a certain tensity (tonus), which is most often measured with palpation, which is usually not objective. This tensity is subject to change in a number of clinical situations, especially in the course of acute or chronic graft rejection, acute tubular necrosis (ATN), inflammatory reactions, etc. First attempts of evaluation of intrarenal pressure were done by Wagner, who performed measurements with use of a thin catheter located constantly during the surgery underneath the transplanted kidney capsule. They demonstrated that in an efficiently functioning organ the subcapsular pressure is usually lower than 15 cm of H20, in acute tubular necrosis it is in the range of 15-40 cm, and in the course of acute graft rejection in exceeds 40 cm.

Salaman and Griffin simplified the measurement technique by using each time a fine aspiration needle connected to manometer. In patients with good and stable kidney function they demonstrated mean intrarenal pressure equal to 27±9,8 mm Hg (around 37 cm H_20), while in patients with acute graft rejection these values were higher and averaged at 51,3 mm Hg (around 70 cm H_20) (1).

Similar measurements were performed in our Centre at the end of 1980s and we used lumbar puncture needles, which after puncturing kidney, were connected to an iv drip line with 0,9 NaCl. The level of stabilized normal saline, after correction for the depth of injected needle, would correspond to the value of intrarenal pressure.

The first, simple device measuring external kidney pressure was developed and patented in 1998 (patent no. 2239687/88. Its action relied on the basis of deflection of dynamometric spring placed in an appropriate casing (draft of the device and measuring method are described in figures 1 and 2).

Figure 1. External view of the first device for measuring external pressure in transplanted kidney.

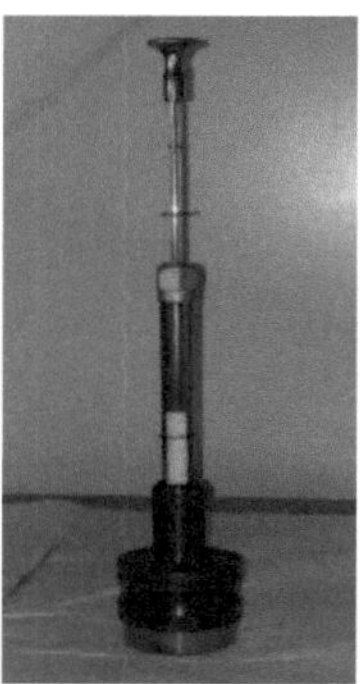

Figure 2.: Scheme of the first tonometer

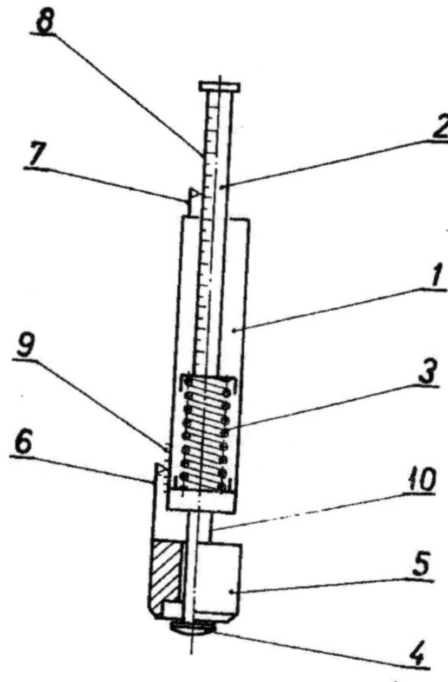

- 1,10. Body of the device
- 2. Trunk of the tonometer with scale
- 3. Spring of the tonometer
- 4. Pressure tip
- 5. Pressure load
- 6. Relative displacement gauge
- 7. Spring deflection gauge
- 8. Piezoelectric sensor
- 9. Electric indicator of pressure force

One end of the spring with pressure tip is based during the measurement on the appropriate point of the abdominal wall above the transplanted kidney. The other end of the spring is pressed with appropriate pressure measured by spring deflection gauge. Depending on hardness and density of the underlying structures, including the kidney graft, different force needs to be used to achieve same displacement (1,5-2 cm) of the abdominal wall. The magnitude of this force is an indirect indicator of existing “tonus” of the transplanted kidney.

Another model of the device was developed in cooperation with RADEX company (engineer Piotr Radion). We named it a renal tonometer and based it on a steering microprocessor and electric converters with feasibility to connect to a computer (scheme of the device, its design and measurement method are presented in figures 3,4,5).

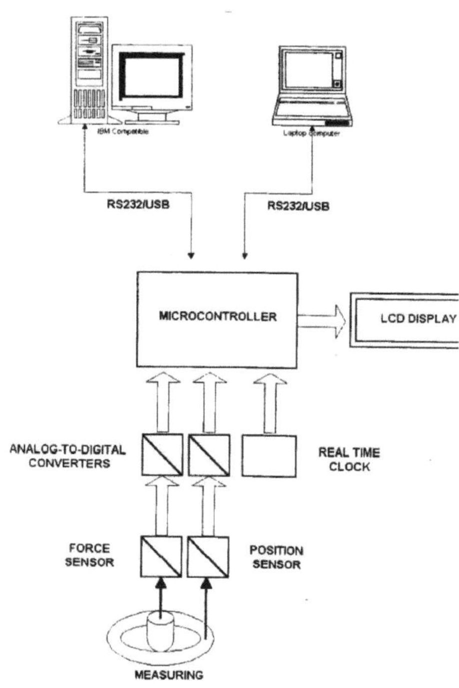

Figure 3. External view of the electronic model of the tonometer

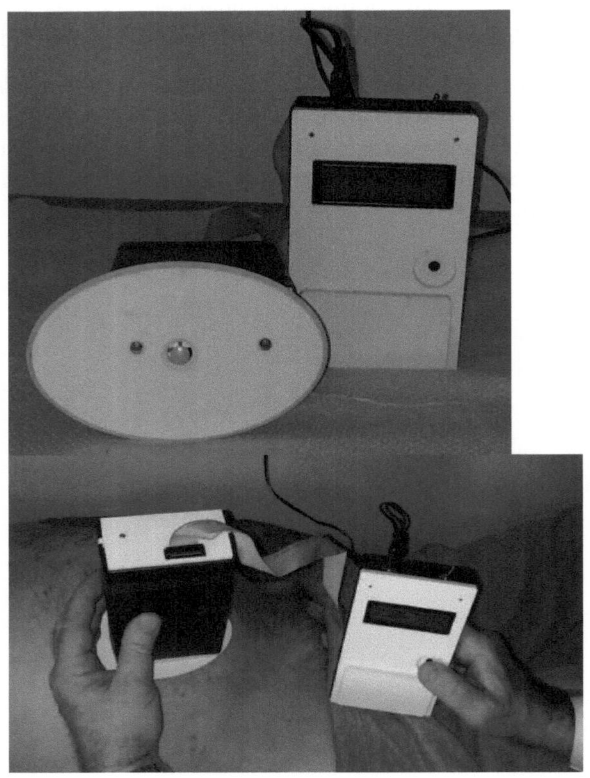

Figure 4/5. Measurement method of external pressure in the transplanted kidney using an electronic version of the tonometer

Altogether we performed 53 measurements in 40 patients (in some patients measurements were repeated accordingly to the condition of the graft). In good and stable kidney function the intrarenal pressure in our patients was at the average 26,5 (14,0 – 45,5) cm H_20, in acute rejection – 63,5 (35-90) cm H_20, in ATN – 34,0 (30-42) cm H_20, and in chronic graft nephropathy – 21,3 (14-42) cm H_20 (5).

We have been using this model for many years. Measurements performed with this device are completely safe, pose no harm to the patient, and can be repeated unlimited number of times. Simplicity of the examination and its bedside feasibility are its additional advantages. In our measurements we pressed abdominal wall with force of 1,5-3,6 kG. We usually performed three measurements and calculated an average of them. During the examination we assured that the patient lies freely on a stable base and the tonometer is placed perpendicular to the abdominal wall. Initially measurements were repeated in the same patient and possible clinical conclusions were drawn from the magnitude of the force necessary to achieve certain assumed deflection of the abdominal wall. And so, for example, if the force necessary to achieve the same deflection was increased by 20-30% or more, it would pose a suspicion about the condition of the graft (possible rejection, pararenal hematoma, urine leak, venous thrombosis, etc.). This examination was, of course, complementary to other routine methods used in such cases (ultrasound, doppler examination, tomography, possible renal biopsy). Our method enabled us to follow and monitor the process of acute graft rejection and its resolution after administered treatment.

The major disadvantage of this method is the difficulty in evaluation of absolute values of results in different patients and comparing them with normal values. This is caused by significant differences in anatomical conditions, thickness of abdominal wall, location and size of the graft between different patients.

The new method of measurement of extrarenal pressure used in our center for several years is based on the difference between force used over the kidney and on the contralateral side of the abdomen with assumed constant deflection of the abdominal wall compared to initial level (around 1,5 cm). This way we have examined 32 patients with kidney grafts in different conditions (fig. 6).

Fig. 6 Comparison of values of tonometric measurements of forces used above the renal graft and contralateral symmetrical side of the abdominal wall.

Patient no	Control group	Acute rejection	Chronic nephropaty
1	0,7	2,1	0,6
2	0,9	1,9	0,5
3	0,7	1,3	0,3
4	0,7	2,0	0,6
5	0,6	0,9	0,6
6	0,6	1,5	0,2
7	0,6	1,6	0,2
8	0,3	2,1	0,3
9	0,4	1,8	0,5
10	0,5	1,5	0,4
11	0,3	2,9	
± SD	0,57 ± 0,18	1,85 ± 0,60	0,42 ± 0,16
	P < 0,001		p < 0,001

Subjects were divided into three groups: controls – with good and stable kidney function (11 persons), acute rejection group (11 persons) and chronic nephropathy group (10 persons). Acute rejection and chronic nephropathy were in most cases verified with biopsy (acute rejection 9 persons, chronic nephropathy 10 persons). In control group with normal kidney function the difference between the force used above the kidney and contralateral symmetrical side of the abdominal wall was 0,57 ± 0,18 kG, in group with acute rejection it was 1,85 ± 0,60 kG, and in chronic nephropathy 0,42 ± 0,16 kG. Differences between control group and group with acute rejection and group with acute nephropathy were statistically significant. Despite the fact that these early results were interesting (especially when it came to differentiating between acute graft rejection and ATN in early postoperative period) and despite we did not note any complications of the measurement, after several years we stopped using this diagnostic method. It was caused by theoretical possibility of bleeding, infection, as well as uncertainty whether the tip of the diagnostic needle actually is in the proper position – and so whether the achieved result is appropriate. Some patients were cautious about their "new kidney" and did not consent to this examination. All these arguments encouraged us to initiate our own diagnostic program of evaluation of external pressure of the transplanted kidney.

We have found no publications of other authors about this diagnostic method in available literature. Significant value is attributed to evaluation of renal graft by ultrasound examination with doppler imaging, especially with evaluation of Resistance Index (RI) or Pulastility Index (PI). According to some authors, RI values above 0,8 with coexistence of other clinical and ultrasonographic features (kidney enlargement, pyramidal edema) can suggest acute graft rejection. (6,7,9). However other publications diminish clinical value of these indices and support the thesis that an elastography examination is a more accurate and modern method of evaluation. This method is based on an ultrasonographic evaluation of tensity and hardness of the examined organ through measurement of velocity of wave propagation. This method gained its advocates in evaluation of mammary glands in women, also in pregnant and lactating mothers, in chronic liver disorders – its results correlate with level of hepatic fibrosis, and recently - in evaluation of renal graft.

Stoch examined patients with acute renal graft rejection (confirmed by biopsy) using method of ARFI (Acoustic Radiation Force Impulse Imaging) – with Siemens Acuson S-2000 device – and demonstrated that mean values of elastography indices were 15% higher compared to the control group.

It seems that the above described noninvasive diagnostic methods could correspond to the below presented methods of evaluation of external pressure although it would require further comparative research in the future.

Nonetheless, the described method of measurement based on differences of pressure forces is not performed simultaneously, which is a certain disadvantage of this diagnostic method. Therefore, a further modification of the renal tonometer was designed with two parallel sensors (measuring probes), which through the configuration of force sensors and analog-to-digital converters would measure the forces and their differences with assumed deflection (by around 1,5-2 cm) over the renal graft and over the symmetrical side of the abdominal wall. (Fig. 7)

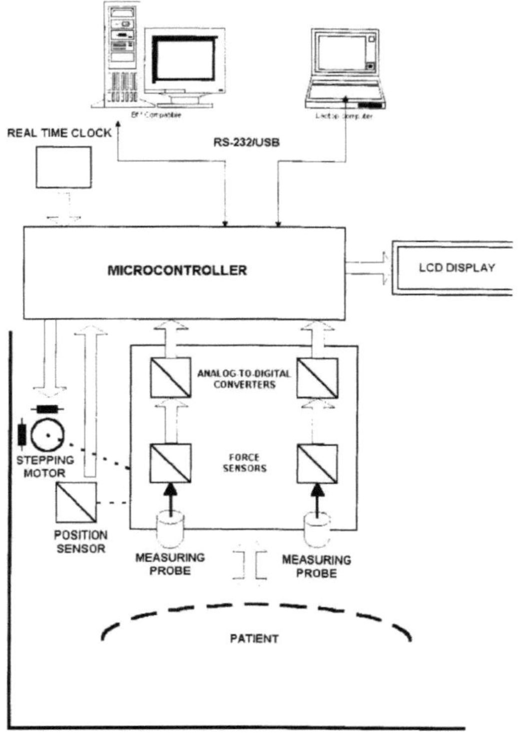

Fig. 7. Scheme of an electronic version of tonometer used for simultaneous measurement of difference in external pressure over the kidney and contralateral, symmetrical side of the abdomen.

These sensors would be placed an appropriate arch mounted to the patient's bed. Their position and tilt angle would be each time adjusted to each patient. Values of used forces and their differences can be displayed or recorded in computer memory. We assume that this method of simultaneous measurements would allow to overcome differences resulting from individual anatomic features of the patient and position of renal grafts, which would make achieved results more objective and valuable.

Pressure measurements of the transplanted kidney, especially extrarenal pressure evaluation with a modified method of examination (measurement of differences in the magnitude of used force (kG) above the kidney and contralateral, symmetrical side of the abdomen) can be a useful complement to currently used noninvasive methods (ultrasound with doppler, elastography) in evaluation of the transplanted kidney.

Our method can have a significant value in differentiating between acute rejection and kidney dysfunction caused by acute tubular necrosis (ATN) in early post -transplantation period.

Chronic nephropathy leads to significant drop of intrarenal pressure in transplanted graft. Confirming this with tonometric examination can support the correct diagnosis

It seems that measurement of extrarenal pressure of the transplanted graft, especially in the above presented modified version, because of its noninvasiveness and ability to repeat the examination multiple times, can have a wider use in the future compared to evaluation of intrarenal pressure.

References:

1. Salaman J.R., Griffin P.J.: Fine-needle internal manometry: a new test for rejection in cyclosporin – treated recipiens of kidney transplants. Lancet 1983,15,2 (8352),709.

2. Wagner E., Pilchmayr R., Wonigeit K.J. et al.: The subcapsular hydrostic pressure of allogenic kidney grafts: a new clinical method for postoperative transplant monitoring. Transplant. Proc. 1983,15,1707.

3. Dziewanowski K., Chłodny J., Bąk L.: Tonometria nerki przeszczepionej – niedoceniana metoda oceny przeszczepu. Nefrol.Dial.Pol.2003,7 (1)28-31.

4. Dziewanowski K.: Renal tonometr. Polish Technical Reviev 1992,1.10.

5. Lapis J., Dziewanowski K.: Manometria wewnątrznerkowa nerki przeszczepionej. Wiad. Lek.1987.XL,20,1379-82.

6. Restrepo-Schafer J.K., Schwerk W.B., Muller T.F.: Intrarenal doppler flow analysis in patients with kidney transplantation and stabile transplant function. Ultraschall.Med. 1999,Jun.20(3),87-92.

7. Covic A., Mardare N., Gusbeth-Tatomir P. et al.: Acute effect of CyA (Neoral) in large artery hemodynamics in renal transplant patients. Kidney Int. 2005, Feb.67(2),732-7.

8. Stock K.F., Klein B.S., Cong M.T. et al.: ARFI-based tissue elasticity quantification and kidney graft dysfunction: first clinical experiences. Clin.Hemorhed.Microcirc. 2011,49, (1-4) 527-35.

9. Kahramans S., Genctoy G., Cill B, et al.: Prediction of renal allograft function with early Doppler ultrasonography. Transplant. Proc.2004,Jun.36(5)1348-51.

10. Castera L., Verginiol J., Foucher J. et al.: Prospective Comparison of Transient Elastography, Fibrotest, APRI, and Liver Biopsy for the Assessment of Fibrosis in Chronic Hepatitis C. Gastroenterology 2005,128,343-50.

11. Sandrin L., Fourquet B., Hasquenoph J.M. e5t al: Transient elasatography: a new noninvasive method for assessment of hepatic fibrosis. Ultrasound in Med.&Biol.2003,29(12) 1705-13.

12. Ziol M., Barget N., Sandrin L. et al.: Correlation between liver elasticity measured by transient elastography and liver fibrosis assessed by morphomanometry in patients with HCV chronic hepatitis. (abstr.) J.Hepatol. 2004;(supl.1)459.

Clinical part.

Parycalcitol + J^{131} - a new route to treatment secondary hyperparathyroidism in patients with chronic kidney disease on long-term dialysis?

Two cases with the dramatic course of secondary hyperparathyroidism in patients with chronic kidney disease on long-term dialysis. Has anything possible been done in management of these patients? Complications associated with impaired bone mineralization among patients with chronic kidney disease on long-term dialysis are observed frequently with an array of pathologic processes being found. Kidney osteodystrophy may be associated with either increased or decreased (adynamic bone disease, osteomalacia, aluminum-induced osteopenia) bone metabolism, as well as mixed forms related to the ß2-microglobulin amyloidosis. Differential diagnosis of various types of osteopathy is difficult and is usually based on the histologic assessment of the bone biopsy. The most typical bone complication in patients with impaired kidney function is osetodistophy with increased bone metabolism, caused by secondary hyperparathyroidism clinically manifesting as osteitis fibrosa. High serum levels of PTH induce osteoclast and osteoblast activity. Early changes, with characteristic increase in the woven osteoid suggesting early, increased osteoplastic bone resorption may be found in a significant percentage of patients with GFR>60 ml/min/1,73 m^2 of the body surface. Lower values of the GFR are associated with both faster bone synthesis and more active resorption with progressive increase in the intraosseous fibrosis and decreased bone mineralization. As the abnormalities progress, which is especially marked in patients on long- term dialysis, a rage of clinical symptoms, such as: severe bone and joint pain, bone deformation, pathological fractures, especially in the spinal region, calcifications of the soft tissues and vessels, including heart valves and lungs. In children, the most common abnormality is growth impairment. In some patient's skin calcifications, with subsequent necrosis, due to increased calcium deposition in small and medium arteries. The diagnosis is based on the typical clinical picture, biochemical parameters (calcium and phosphate ratio, parathormone levels, characteristic radiologic charges and sometimes, bone histology. Prevention and treatment of these complications includes effective dialysis, appropriate low-phosphate diet with limitation of the protein supply to the 0.8 g/kg of the body mass, adequate calcium and active Vitamin D3 supply, introduction of the phosphate binding medications (sevelamer or lantan) as well as calcimimetic use (substances activating parathyroid gland calcium receptors inhibiting both its up-regulation and PTH secretion). In the severe cases, with insufficient effect of the treatment described above, parathyroidectomy is required after close ultrasound and scintigraphy-based assessment of these glands. However, even such treatment may be insufficient in some cases, as presented below.

CASE REPORTS

Her we would like to present two cases of the extremely advanced hyperparathyroidism with high bone turnover and dramatic course over the period of long-term follow-up. In both, despite multidirectional treatment, the outcome of the therapy proved unsuccessful.

Case I

Patient M.H., born in 1951, under care of our center since February 1992, since the diagnosis of the chronic glomerulonephritis with nephrotic syndrome in the stadium of the kidney insufficient (creatinine levels of 1.8 mg/dL with normal calcium and phosphate levels). Kidney biopsy has never been performed in this patient, so no histologic data is available. In the treatment steroids and azathioprine was used, however without complete remission. Since 1993 in the treatment non-steroid anti-inflammatory drugs were introduced and angiotensin converting enzyme inhibitors – no improvement in the kidney function parameters was noted. Throughout the entire period of follow-up, the patient was treated with calcium carbonate and alphadiol. No monitoring of the parathyroid hormone levels was performed. In June 1997, in the routine abdominal ultrasound scan the tumor of the left kidney was found with subsequent nephrectomy.

In histopathology from the excised material two neoplasms were found to be present in the kidney: stadium I carcinoma clalocellulare and stadium II carcinoma papillare. After a surgery the clinical progression of the kidney insufficiency was observed (creatinine levels - 3 mg/dLm GFR of 23ml/min). Patient's and mental condition worsened significantly, with notable mood disorder (depression), negative attitude to further diagnostics and treatment. In the late December 2000 the patient was re-admitted with the end-stage kidney failure with necessity for the urgent hemodialysis. When hemodialysed, the patient was largely non-adherent, with poor compliance to the dietary and water restrictions, often presenting with hypervolemia. Moreover, she did not consent for the kidney transplantation. In the treatment, except for the hypotensive drugs the calcium and vitamin D3 supplements were used (Alphadiol 0,25ug and Calperos 3g/day). In July 2003 the PTH levels were 856 pg/ml. In the thyroid ultrasound the enlarged parathyroid gland in the area of the upper part of the left thyroid lobe (mean diameter of 6,3 mm) was noted. Further diagnostics (scintigraphy) or treatment (surgery) was not performed, due to the lack of patient's consent. The wasting progressed, with the loss of 15 kg of the body mass with pains in the region of the thoracic and lumbar spine. Patient's posture changed notably – kyphosis became apparent. The patient continued to object to the surgery of the parathyroid adenoma, moreover she refused in-hospital treatment for initiation of calcimimetics and Renagel. In February 2009, chest computed tomography was performed; in the scans of the lower part of the neck enlarged thyroid gland was seen. In the right thyroid lobe calcified masses of the 0.5 and 0.9 cm diameter were recorded, while in the left lower the focal lesion of 0.6 cm was observed. In the left lung the nodule (0.4 cm) was seen, with no enlarged lymph nodes in the pulmonary hilar regions nor in the mediastinum. In the CT scan result multiple lesions in the ribs (distortions with regenerative reaction) which may be associated with the rib fractures. Additionally, lesions in the vertebral bodies (Th8-L1), described as possible post-osteoporotic fractures, were found.

Patient consistently refused to consent for the surgery of the parathyroid adenoma. In 2009 treated with Mimpara and Ranagel, but with no clinical or biochemical improvement (PTH above 3000 pg/ml, phosphates within the normal range). The patient died in October 2009 due to the progressive heart and respiratory failure.

Case II.

Patient S.I., female, born in 1953with right kidney excised in 1959 due to the hydronephrosis with chronic left-sided pyelonephritis (1973) which progressed to the kidney failure ten years later. In 1985 the dialysis was introduced with kidney transplantation performed in May that year which functioned poorly and was removed in July of the same year. The hyperparathyroidism was observed during the follow-up, with thyroid gland resection and one-sided parathyroidectomy in February 1992 and later the same year the second parathyroidectomy. The excision was guided by the ultrasound scanning and the scintigraphy in both cases. In the early 90-ties we did not routinely assess the parathyroid hormone levels. In April 2002 PTH level was 2150 pg/ml (the first result ever), with calcium and phosphate levels within the normal range. In the ultrasound scan of the neck, in the right thyroid stump the nodule, described as probable parathyroid gland, was found. This finding resulted in the next, third parathyroidectomy. It did not effect in the significant decrease of the PTH levels (500 pg/ml). Osteoporosis was clinically apparent with pathological bilateral fracture of the femoral necks which necessitated implantation of the hip prostheses (firstly right-side, then the left one). At that time PTH levels were 1500 pg/ml and increased to above 2000 pg/ml in 2006. In the CT scan of the neck and chest the contrast enhancing nodule, sized 23x15 mm in the frontal mediastinum was observed, accompanied by the disseminated, characteristic for the hyperparathyroidism osteolytic lesion in the ribs, and the dense fluid in the sternoclavicular joints, more pronounced on the right. In scintigraphy the mediastinal tumor was confirmed and in June 2006 the patient was transferred to the department of General, Vascular and Transplant Surgery, Medical University, Warsaw, where she underwent the excision of the lesion (fourth parathyroidectomy). After tumor excision the PTH levels dropped to almost 300 pg/ml, however in September 2006 the levels of PTH rose again (above value of 1500 pg/ml) with normal calcium and phosphate serum levels. The patient underwent treatment with Mimpara 9300 mg/day then 60 mg/day). In December 2006 the patient died due to progressive vascular-respiratory disorder in the mechanism similar to the patient described as the first case.

Two case histories of our patients indicate, that despite full access to the modern medical care in some cases medics remain helpless in the respect of the inhibition of the progression of the secondary hyperparathyroidism in such patients.

Calcimimetics remain a fairly efficient treatment option, however its efficacy, despite often high does, is limited to PTH not exceeding 1000 pg/ml. With higher levels of parathyroid hormone, the treatment of choice is parathyroidectomy. The clinical situation becomes even more complicated when the patient refuses to consent for the operation, or when the functions of the removed parathyroid glands are taken by the ectopic focuses (as noted in one of our patients). Theoretically we could consider if the co-administration of Cynacalcet with isotope (e.g. J^{131}) would be helpful in such cases. Cynacacet, as the carrier with affinity to the calcium receptors, mainly in parathyroid glands, while J131 as the isotope inducing its involution. Such an association might be also used in other parathyroid pathologies (e.g. primary cancer of this gland)

The problem is also associated to the oral form of Cynacalcet which is available currently, as well as to the fact that calcium receptors are located also, however in minor quantities, in other tissues. This is the reason why at the moment such a co-administration is safe. However, it seems that the concept might be clinically tired, after adequate consent and cooperation with Amgen, which is the current owner and distributor of the Cynacalcet. In the last years another medication used for the prevention and treatment of the secondary parathyroid in patients with chronic kidney disease became available (parycalcytol – Zempler manufactured by Abbott). This drug is selectively activation the vitamin D receptors (VDR) in parathyroid glands, with no influence of the VDR in the gut. It is used by intravenous injection, perhaps co-administration of such a medication with J^{131} would be more real and beneficial for the patients, than J^{131}-cynacalcet administration. This would certainly require the adequate synthesis of the new co-formulation and a clinical trial.

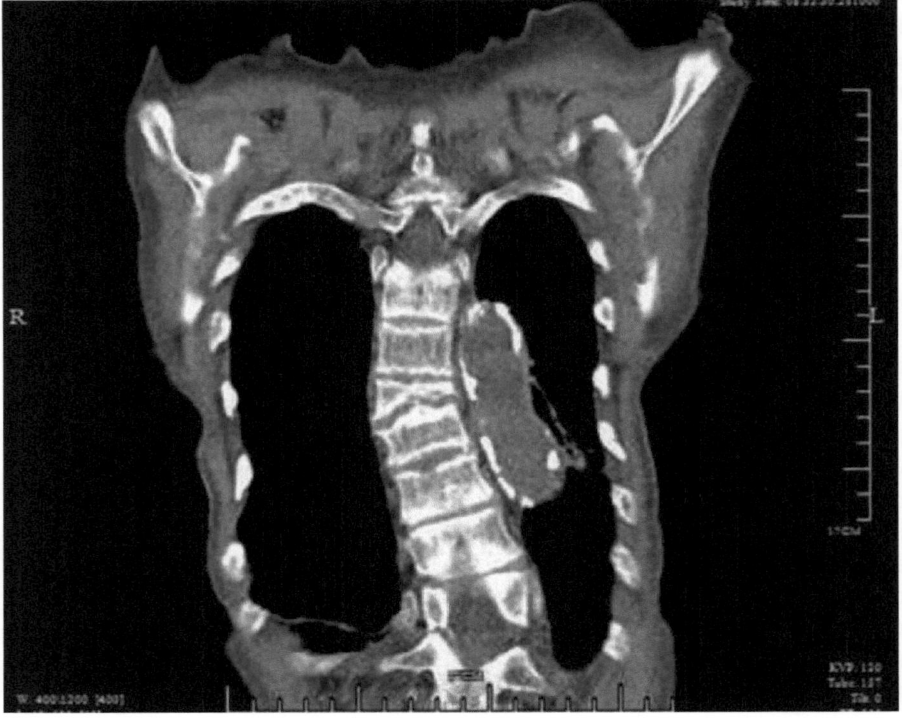

Case .1

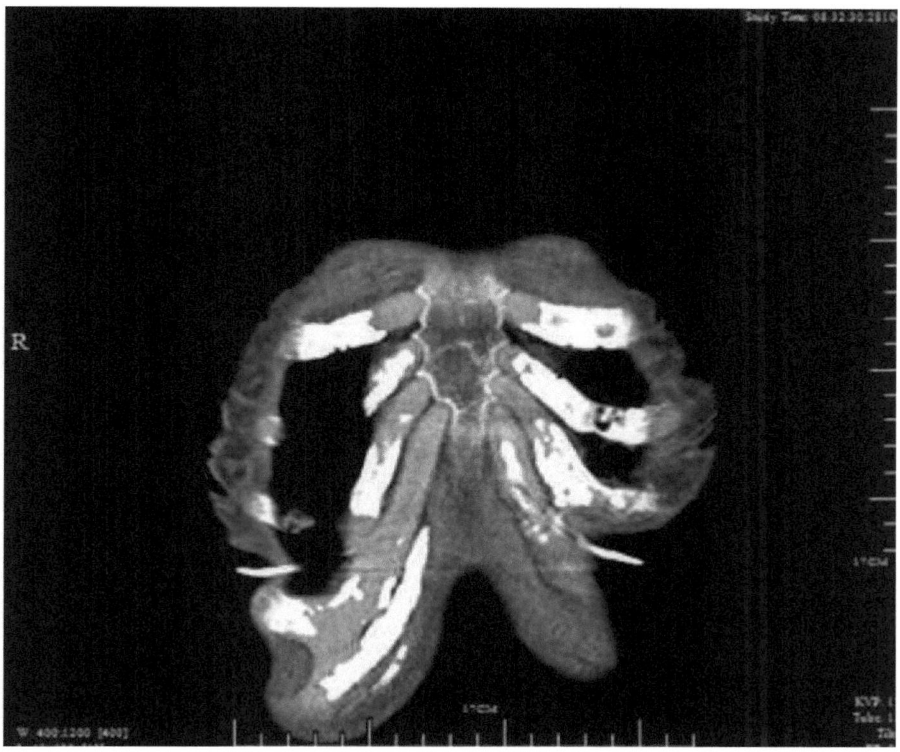

Case 2.

References:

1.Brancaccio D., Cozzolino M., Cannela G et all: Secondary Hyperparathyroidism in Chronic Dialysis Patients: Results of the Italian FARO Survey on Treatment and Mortality. Blood Purif. 2011 May 28: 32(2): 124

2. Cunningham J, Locatelli F, Rodriguez M:.Secondary hyperparathyroidysm pathogenesis, disease progression and therapeutic options. Clin J Am Soc Nephrol. 2011 Apr. 6(4):913.

3. Czekalski S., Oko A., Pawlaczyk K, i wsp.: Przewlekła nierwydolność nerek - aktualne metody hamowania progresji. Pol. Arch. Med. Wewn. 2004, CXI, 97.

4. DruekeT., Martin D., Rodriguez M.: Can calcimimetics inhibit parathyroid hyperplasia? Evidence from preclinical studies. Nephrol.Dial.Transplant. 2007,22,1828.

5. Maberti F., Saha H., Neyer U. et al.: The Pan-European ECHO Study Investigator Group K/DOQI target achievement is improved with cinacalcet (Mimpara/Sensipar) in clinical practice. Presented et: European Renal Association, European Dialysis and Transplantation Association (ERA-EDTA) XLV Congress; May 10-13,2008; Stocholm, Sweden.

6. Melamed ML., EustaceJA., Plantinga L. et al.: Changes in serum calcium, phosphate, and PTH and the risk of death in incident dialysis patients: alongitudinal study. Kidney Int. 2006,70,351.

7. Messa P., Macario F., Yaqoob M. et al.: The OPTIMA Study: assessing a new cinacalcet (Sensipar/Mimpara) treatment algorithm for secundary hyperparathyroidism. Clin. J. Am.Soc. Nephrol. 2008;3,36.

8. Locatelli F., Cannata-Andia J.B., Drueke T.B. et all: Managment of disturbances of calcium and phosphate metabolism in chronic renal insufficiency, with emphasuis on the control of hyperphosphatemia, Nephrol. Dial. Transplant. 2002, 17, 723

Immunosuppression on kidney transplantation among identical twins – yes or not?

A case of successful kidney transplantation among two homozygous twins is presented here. Prior to the familiar kidney transplantation from the identical twins the patient underwent peritoneal and hemodialysis as well as cadaveric kidney transplant from an unrelated donor. In this patient vascular accessibility was poor and the second, familiar transplantation was performed urgently. Transplanted kidney function proved excellent, however the issues of the best immunosuppressant to be selected are under consideration. Decision on the use or withdrawal of immunosuppressant drugs requires careful revive of the disease status, concomitant disease and factors influencing the final outcome.

The era of kidney transplantation has begun on the 23rd of December 1954 in Boston, after successful procedure between identical twins performed by Joseph Murray. The transplant recipient survived for 9 years without immunosuppressive therapy and died on the heart infarction. Successful transplantation among twins have prompted further attempts for such a treatment also among unrelated individuals. However, due to the immunological barrier the failure rate was high – the regular kidney transplantation programmed, also from unrelated donors, was initiated in 1954 after introduction of Azathioprine and Prednisolone to the immunosuppressive treatment. In the next years the understanding of mechanisms of immunological response has led to notable increase of pharmacological immunotherapy availability. Contemporary immune suppressive regiments have extended the mean transplant survival time in Poland 8-10 years. Transplantation between the closely related individuals, especially homozygous twins, seems to be a different issue in this context. Opinions on the immunosuppressant therefore drug toxicity might be avoided. However, it was noted that risk of recurrence of the primary disease, which might have been treated with immune suppression is high. Moreover, it was observed that during the intrauterine fetus growth DNA mutation is often observed, resulting in phenotypic and genotypic divergence even in homozygous twins.

These facts lead to variety in opinions on the therapeutic approach in such cases. In this work we would like to describe the case of the transplantation in homozygous twins and related clinical dilemmas.

In this report, we would like to present the case of 29-year-old male. Caucasian patient with stage 5 chronic kidney disease due to diarrhea related hemolytic-uremic syndrome in the childhood (7th month of life, treated with temporary peritoneal dialysis). The patient was dialyzed since 1996, at first by peritoneal dialysis, then due to the recurrent peritonitis and loss of exchange efficacy, with hemodialysis. One year later (12.03.1997) the first kidney transplantation was performed with the organ harvested from the cadaveric donor (HLA mismatch (MM) 3, kidney from 18 years old male, Caucasian donor, PRA antibody activity - 0%). Hemodialysis was reintroduced after the graft function impairment (chronic graft nephropathy) in 2003. Hemodialysis, despite every effort for maximum optimization, was poorly tolerated by the patients. Difficulties with blood pressure normalization, secondary hyperparathyroidism and concomitant osteopathy were observed. The patient underwent two surgeries of the pathological thoracic spine fractures and splenectomy due to spontaneous splenic rupture and bleeding.

The difficulty on the maintenance of the permanent vascular line for hemodialysis was notable. Several attempts to create the arteriovenous fistulae failed, with necessity to use carotid, subclavian and ultimately femoral venous catheters. After voluntary assent, the second kidney transplantation was performed with kidney harvested from monozygotic twin, after confirmation of the full genetic concordance, on 26.10,2009. Prior to this procedure PRA activity was monitored closely, with increase to 50% after loss of the first graft and subsequent total loss of reactivity (0%) before the second transplantation. Anti-HLA antibody level was not monitored.

In the postsurgical period the deep venous thrombosis was observed as well as urinary retention in bladder related to the urethral stenosis. After introduction of antibiotics, anticoagulants, distending of the urethra all the above symptoms resolved. The patient was discharged after 21 days with excellent kidney function (copious dieresis, serum creatinine levels of 0,72 mg/dl, GFR – 137,5 ml/min) and has been regularly followed up ever since. The remaining kidney function in the donor is satisfactory as well, with transient increase in blood pressure only and good renal function (creatinine – 1,2mg/dl, GFR – 80ml/min).

The immunosuppressive therapy in this case was challenging from the outset. The patient had been on kidney replacement treatment for 13 years in total (peritoneal and hemodialysis: two renal transplantations) with loss of vascular accessibility and severe treatment complications (hyperparathyroidism and osteopathy necessitated urgent transplantation). The fact that DNA testing confirmed genotypic identity between donor and recipient, as well as the primary disease – HUS being contraindication for calcineurin inhibitor use, favored immunosuppressant withdrawal. On the other hand, possibility of the immunization during the first transplantation and necessity to reduce the risk after the second procedure (high fatality rate associated with poor vascular access) prompted for cautious use of immunosuppressant.

All in all, the patient has received the reduced dose of steroids (methylprednisone infusions – 250mg q.d. i.v./3 days with subsequent oral prednisone 20mg daily in decreasing doses) and mofetil mycophenolate 1g b.i.d. Due to the DVT history occasional anticoagulant and antibiotic treatment was commenced. Further reduction of the immune suppression is currently being considered.

Reference data remain inconclusive in the respect of practical management of such a patient. Kessaris in large analysis of outcome in 120 cases of kidney transplantation from twins in the USA and 12 in UK, performed from 1988-2004 have shown that the success rate in such procedures is high. In the USA one and five year transplant survival rates were 99,17% and 88,96%, respectively. However, in this study is not clear if twin identity was always confirmed by DNA testing or was largely phenotype based. Moreover comparative analysis of the treatment results in kidney transplanted twins on immune suppression (n=82) and without it (n=38) and without it (n=38) did not produce conclusive data (differences statistically insignificant p=0,12). In the five year follow-up in the group on immunosuppression 4 individuals lost the kidney, and two died, while in the non-treated group 5 patients lost graft and 1 died.

Sanchez-Escuredo in analysis in five patients with kidney grafts from their monozygotic twins shown that kidney transplantation from living monozygotic twin is associated to outstanding clinical outcomes. Immunosuppression therapy to suppress alloimmune response in probably unnecessary 11 zygosity has been confirmed.

To sum up, the presented data do not allow to select the optimal treatment in the similar clinical situations. Individual consideration must include degree of genetic and immunologic concordance, concomitant disease, as well as additional factors influencing future outcome of the transplantation (age, gender, number of transplantation) with decision on the exact immunosuppressive regimen related also to the function transplanted kidney.

References:

1. Bentley FR., Sutherland DE., Fred DS. et al.: Similar renal allograft functional survival rates for kidneys from sibling donors matched for zero-versus-one haplotype with the recipient. Transplantation 1984, Dec:38(6),674-679.

2. Day E., Kearns PK., Taylor C.J. et al.: Transplantation between monozygotic twins: how identical are they? Transplantation 2014 Sep.98(5),485-489.

3. Gumprich M., Woeste G., Kohlhaw K. et al.: Living Related Kidney Transplantation Between Identical Twins. Transplant. Proc. 2002,34,2205-2206.

4. Kaufman DB., Sutherland DE., Noreen H. et al.: Renal transplantation between living-related sibling pairs matched for zero-HLA haplotypes. Transplantation 1989 Jan 47(1),113-119.

5. Kessaris N., Mukherjee D., Chandak P. et al.: Renal Transplantation in Identical Twins in United States and United Kingdom. Transplantation 2008,86,1572-1577.

6. Krishnan N., Buchanan PM., Dzebisashvili N. et al.: Monozygotic transplantation: concerns and opportunities. Am J Transplant. 2008, Nov. 8(11),2343-2351.

7. Pszenny A., Gutowska D., Czerwiński J. et al.: Long-term survival after kidney transplantation from homozygotic twin – a case report. Ann Transplant. 2007, 12(1),46-48.

8. Mattos AM., Bennett WM., Barry JM. Et al.: HLA-identical sibling renal transplantation 21-yr single –center experience. Clin Transplant. 1999 Apr. 13(2),158-167.

9. Matas AJ., Payne WD., Sutherland DE. Et al.: 2500 living donor kidney transplants: a single-center experience. Ann Surg. 2001 Aug., 234(2),149-164.

10. Rao Z., Huang Z., Song T. et al.: A lesson from kidney transplantation among identical twins: Case report and literature review. Transpl.Immunol. 2015 Sept.33(1),27-29.

11. Sanchez-Escuredo A., Barijas A., Revuelta I. et al.: Kidney transplantation from living monozygotic twin donor with no maintenance immunosuppression. Nefrologia 2015, 35(4),358-362.

12. Shimmura H., Tanabe K., Ishida H. et al.: Long-term results of living kidney transplantation from HLA identical sibling donors under calcineurin inhibitor immunosuppression. Int J Urol.2006 May,13(5),502-508.

13. Simmons RL., van Hook EJ., Yunis eJ. et al.: 100 sibling kidney transplants followed 2 to 7 ½ years: a multifactorial analysis. Ann Surg.1977 Feb.185(2),196-204.

14. Sumrani N., Delaney V., Ding ZK. et al.: HLA-identical renal Transplants: impact of cyclosporine on intermediate-term survival and renal function, Am J Kidney Dis. 1990 Nov. 16(5),417-422.

15. Yong Kyun Kim, Hye Eun Yoon, Su Hyun Kim et al.: Long-term follow-up of three identical twin transplant recipients without maintenance immunosuppressive therapy. Nephrology 2008,13,447-449.

Necessity of monitoring of the drug level (Mycophenolate Mofetil) in blood a patients after kidney transplantation.

Wide introduction of calcineurin inhibitors in transplantation since the 1980s resulted in a significant improvement in survival of both transplants and patients. However, when we use these and other immunosuppressive drugs we constantly have to achieve balance between the need to protect the patient against rejection and the potential toxicity of these medications. In extreme cases we can even speak of the so-called "immunosuppressive disease" which results from multiple adverse effects of these drugs affecting multiple organs and causing disorders such as arterial hypertension, diabetes, bone marrow toxicity, predispositions to cancer and infections, as well as acute or chronic nephrotoxicity. Therefore, modern transplantology commonly recommends monitoring of blood levels of the most commonly used immunosuppressive drugs. This applies to both calcineurin inhibitors (cyclosporine, tacrolimus, Advagraf) as well as mTOR inhibitors (Sirolimus, Everolimus). During the use of monoclonal (OKT3) and polyclonal antibodies (ATG, Thymoglobulin), it is necessary to check leukocytosis, and more preferably, the level of CD3 lymphocytes (decrease in the number of these cells during treatment should not exceed more than 50-100/mm^3 of blood). Among clinicians there is a discussion whether levels of mycophenolate mofetil (MMF) or even mycophenolate sodium (MPS) should be routinely monitored. Therefore, we would like to present our initial experience with this issue. Large individual variability in metabolism of calcineurin inhibitors forced the need to monitor their blood levels in patients undergoing organ transplantation. Most of the centers assess the so-called C_0 level - that is the concentration of the drug at 12 hours after of administration. Determination of the so-called C_0 (that is the drug concentration at 2 hours after administration) is less accepted due to the lower reliability of the data received. Assessment of area under the curve of drug levels is not as widespread because of problems with its practical use, and because of the costs. Concentration of CyA can be assessed both in serum and whole blood. The used methods are: HPLC - high flow chromatography (high performance liquid chromatography), EMIT (enzyme multiplied immunoassay technique) or FPIA (fluorescence polarization immunoassay). MEIA (Microparticle Enzyme Immunoassay) is the most commonly used method to assess the concentration of tacrolimus, and it is based on the determination of monoclonal antibodies in automated analyzers. Recommended concentration levels of drug in the blood of these patients are dependent on the time period after the transplantation as well as the applied research methodology. For example, in the initial phase after transplantation, C_0 of CyA should be 250-450 ng/ml, and after a few months, about 150 ng/ml (FPIA method). The similar applies to concentration of C_2 – initial values should be 1.5-2 mg/ml, and later 0.8 to 1.0 ug / ml. Recommended levels of tacrolimus (C_0) for the initial dose of 0.15 mg/kg/day in the early period after transplantation should be in the range of 10-20 ng / ml, and after a few months between 5-7 ng / ml. Determination of the AUC involves adding up the drug blood levels in a number of samples taken within a few hours after ingestion. It is emphasized that there are significant differences between absolute values of measurements of the original drug concentration compared to its generic formulations. Recommended blood level of mTOR inhibitors is within range of 5-25 ng/d using HPLC method. It is emphasized in the literature that combination of these drugs with calcineurin inhibitors should be used with extreme caution because both these groups of medications are metabolized by the same cytochrome in liver (P-450 III A cytochrome).

In our center, since April 2016, we have conducted plasma level MPA analysis performing enzyme immunoassay EMIT method using a homogeneous enzyme immunoassay technique. These tests were conducted on an analyzer produced by Siemens based on the principle of competition for binding sites of MPA- antibodies MPA present in the sample competes with the MPA labeled with an enzyme, glucose-6-phosphate dehydrogenase (G6PHD). Active, unbound form of the enzyme converts nicotinamide adenine dinucleotide (NAD) into an antibody (a substrate for NADH), which results in a change of absorption which can be measured spectrophotometrically. Since the enzyme activity decreases after binding with the antibody, it allows to measure concentration of MPA in the sample. Using this research method, we have performed 23 AUC tests (with three samples of blood for each of them) in 21 patients until now. The graph depicting measured values is presented below.

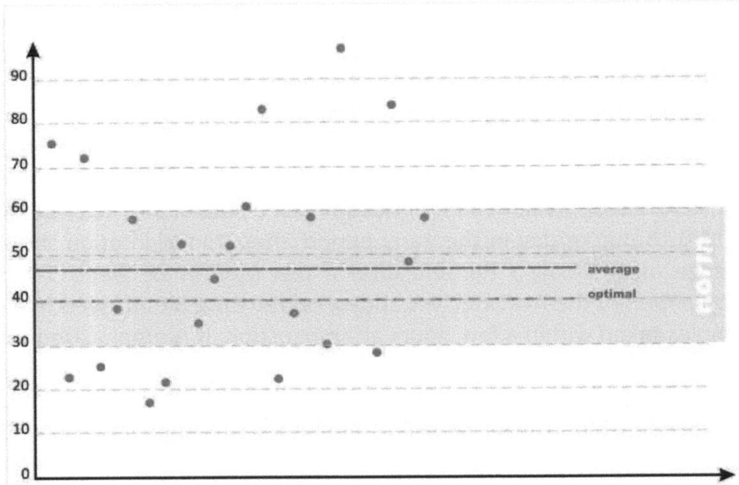

Fig1. Mean levels of MMF in patients' blood (mg.h/L) achieved with assessment of area under curve (AUC) - values obtained in each case from three blood samples

The average assessed value of AUC was 46.96 ± 21.98 (recommended AUC is 30-60 mg.h / L, the optimal is 40 mg.h / L). In several cases the AUC values differed far from the recommended range, which resulted in correction of drug dose. In one case of highly increased AUC (75 mg.h / L), the patient developed symptoms of CMV infection and we believe that a significant reduction in the dose of MMF facilitated prompt control of this infection.

Assessment of blood levels of mycophenolate mofetil (particularly the most commonly used formulation mycophenolate mofetil) is still controversial. A number of transplant centers routinely use the manufacturer's recommended dose of 2 g/day (2x1,0g) in adult patients, at most modifying it according to the weight of the patient or dividing daily dose into 3-4 doses in case gastrointestinal adverse effects occur. However, an increasing number of clinical studies and literature reports criticize such mode of treatment. They believe that a number of adverse effects of this drug can result from an uncontrolled increase of its level in blood despite administration of a recommended dose. Also, greater frequency and severity of graft rejection may in some cases be the result of a low level of drug in the blood despite the typical dosage. There are at least two methods of monitoring blood levels of this drug. The first involves determining the concentration of mycophenolic acid in the blood MPA C_0 immediately before the next dose. This is a simple way, requiring only a single blood draw. The recommended level of MPA C_0 when it is administered in combination with CyA is 1,3mg / and, when MMF is co-administered with tacrolimus, it is 1.9 mg / L. However, a disadvantage of this method is a low correlation of obtained C_0 values with area under the curve (AUC). Therefore, it is currently preferred to use a three-point assessment system, that is determination of drug concentration in the blood at 20 min, 1 hour and 3 hours after administration. It is assumed that the recommended aggregate values of mycophenolate mofetil levels assessed by this method should be in the range of 30 - 60 mg.h / L, taking into account that different values are necessary in patients co-treated with CyA or tacrolimus. Currently there are big difficulties in developing a practical method for monitoring the level of mycophenolate sodium (MPS) which becomes more increasingly used in transplantation centers because of intolerance of mycophenolate mofetil caused by gastrointestinal adverse effects in some patients. These difficulties arise from the fact that the administration of mycophenolate mofetil is followed by an almost immediate release of this drug in the gastrointestinal tract, while in the case of mycophenolate sodium (MPS) this process is delayed which may partly be due to different individual rate of gastric emptying. It is further complicated by widespread use of proton pump inhibitors which can cause premature dissolution of the tablets and faster release of the active drug. It is attempted to solve this problem by monitoring blood levels of the drug at 3 and 4 hours after ingestion. Currently, clinical trials are performed in order to develop optimal assay method.

Conclusions

The above review of the literature, clinical trials and our initial experience suggest clearly that monitoring the levels of immunosuppressive drugs, especially after kidney transplantation, is a necessity. It seems that this also applies in selected cases to monitoring blood levels of mycophenolate mofetil, which is reflected by an increasing use of these assays in transplantation centers.

References:

1. Sabatini S., Ferguson R.M., Helderman J.H., et al.: Drug substitution in transplantation: a National Kidney Foundation white paper. Am. J.Kidney Dis. 1999,33,389-393.

2. Bodziak K., Hrick D.: Minimizing the side effects of immunosuppression in kidney transplant recipients. Transplantation 2003,8,160-165.

3. KDIGO Clinical Practice Guideline for Care of Kidney Transplant Recipients. Am. J. Transplant. 2009,9, supl.3.

4. Durlik M. Rowiński W.: Zalecenia dotyczące leczenia immunosupresyjnego po przeszczepieniu narządów unaczynionych. Fundacja Zjednoczeni dla Transplantacji. Warszawa. Grudzień 2012.

5. Gil J.S., Tonelli M.,MixC.etal.:Theeffectofmaintenanceimmunosuppression medication on the change in kidney allograft function. Kidney Int. 2004,65,692-694.

6.KanmazT.,KnechtleS.:Novelagentsorstrategiesforimmunosuppressionafter renal transplantation. Transplantation 2003,8,172-175.

7. Perico N., Ruggenenti P., Gotti E. et al.: In renal transplantation blood cyclosporine levels soon after surgery act as major determinant of rejection: insight from M.Y.S.S. trial. Kidney Int.2004,65,1084-1090.

8. Meier-Kriesche HU., LiS.,GruessnerR.W.etal.:Immunosuppression:Evolution in practice and trends. 1994-2004 Am. J.Transplant. 2006,6 (2),1111-1131.

9. Doyle I., Zikri A.M., Bennett W.E. I wsp. Area under the curve (AUC) bioequivalence (BE) of mycophenolate mofetil (MMF): CellCept vs generic. Abstract presented at the American Society of Nephrology. Renal Week 2010. Denver 16-21.11.2010.

10. Kunicki P.K., Pawiński T.: Równoważność biologiczna preparatów generycznych leków immunosupresyjnych – różnice farmakokinetyczne i konsekwencje dla terapii monitorowej stężenia leku. Nefrol.Dial.Pol. 2012 (4) 181-186.

11. Yang C.W.,Ahn H.J., Kim W.Y. et al.: Cyclosporine withdrawal and mycophenolate mofetil treatment effects on the progression of chronic cyclosporine nephrotoxicity. Kidney Int.2002.62(1), 20-30.

12. Figurski M.J. Nawrocki A., Pescovitz M.D. et al.: Development of a predictive limited sampling strategy for estimation of mycophenolic acid area under the

concentration time curve in patients receiving concomitant sirolimus or cyclosporine. Ther Drug Monit. 2008,30,445-455.

13. Mendez R., Gowna T., Yang H.C. et al.: A prospective, randomized trial of tacrolimus in combination with sirolimus or mycophenolate mofetil in kidney transplantation: Results at 1 year. Transplantation 2005,80,303-309.

14.Pawiński T.: Terapeutyczne monitorowanie stężenia kwasu mykofenolowego w terapii immunosupresyjnej – zalecenia I wątpliwości. Reaktywacja.2010,3,13-15.

15. de Jonge H., Naesens M., Kuypers D.R.: New Insights into the Pharmacokinetic and Pharmacodynamics of the Calcineurin Inhibitors and Mycophenolic acid: possible consequences for therapeutic drug monitoring in solid organ transplantation. Ther Drug Monit. 2009,31,416-435.

16. Kees M.G., Steinke T., Moritz S. et al.: Omeprazole Impairs the Absorption of Mycofenolate Mofetil but not of Mycofenolate Sodium in Healthy Volunteers. J.Clin. Pharmacol. 2011.Sep. 8.

17. Sommerer C., Muller-Krebs S., Schaier M i et al.: Pharmacokinetic and pharmacodynamics analysis of enteric-coated mycophenolate sodum: limited sampling strategies and clinical outcome in renal transplant patients. Br. J..Clin. Pharmacol. 2010,69,346-357.

18. Arens W. ,Bruer S., Choudhury S. et al.: Enteric-Coated Mycophenolate sodum delivers bioequivalent MPA exposure compared with mycophenolate mofetil. Clin.Transpl. 2005,19,199-206.

19. Cooper M., Salvadori M., Budde K.: Leczenie immunosupresyjne z użyciem powlekanych tabletek dojelitowych mycofenolatu sodu u pacjentów po przeszczepieniu nerki: skuteczność I dawkowanie. Transplantation Rev. 2012,26,233-240.

20. Salvadori M., Bertoni E., Budde K. et al.: Superior efficacy of enteric-coated mycophenolate vs mycophenolate mofetil in de novo transplant recipients: pooled analysis. Transplant. Proc. 2010,42,1325-1328.

Kidney transplantation – our experience.

According to various authors, the mean time of kidney graft survival ranges from 8 to 12 years . These results have recently improved for different reasons: better diagnostic methods, effective and prompt treatment of post – transplant complications and modern immunosuppressive regimens. Even better results can be achieved in kidneys transplanted from live donors which is explained by maximal shortening of cold ischemia time (CIT) and good immunologic compatibility.

Therefore, it is interesting to present results from our own center, where kidney transplantation has begun in 1982. Since then we have obtained 99% of kidney grafts from deceased donors with beating hearts. We have only performed less than twenty kidney transplantations from live donors including several grafts obtained with laparoscopy. This situation was caused by multiple factors, including lack of definite and unforced consent of our patients' families and the opinion of our transplantation team that we should first obtain organs from deceased donors without putting potential living donors at risk of early and late complications of nephrectomy. This view is concordant with official statement of WHO and guidelines of Convention on Human Rights and Biomedicine from Oviedo, year 1997 (principle of subsidiarity).

In our centre, after a year from transplantation, a mean of 94% of kidney grafts are functioning. Currently we manage about 420 transplanted patients and some additional patients are lost to follow-up because they moved to other transplantation centers. In this observed group there are 75 patients 15 years or more after transplantation, including 28 patients with stable and functioning grafts 20 years or more after transplantation as well as 3 patients with a functioning graft after 28, 28 , and 29 years respectively.

Results and their analysis

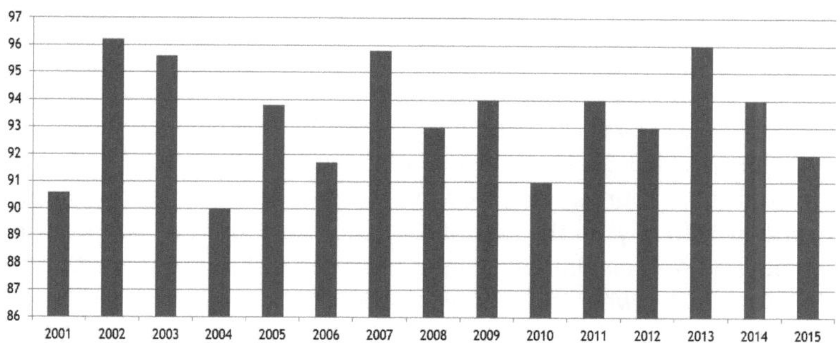

Fig. 1. One –year survival, expressed in percentage, of kidney grafts obtained from dead donors in our Centre in years 2001-2015

Fig.2. Summary of long-term survival of transplanted kidneys in Centre of Transplantology in Regional Hospital in Szczecin

No.	Mean time of graft functioning (in years)	Age of recipient	Age of donor	Sex compatibility: present M/F	Sex compatibility: absent M_D/F_R	Sex compatibility: absent F_D/M_R	Non-compatibility in HLA points (average)	PRA% patients	CIT [h]	Main disease of the donor
75 M50 W25	17.8±5,51	34±11.76	37±11.76	45	21	9	15.1p 2.83 antyg.	0-3%→54 7-20%→13 >20%→8	3-45 19.6 ±8.81	GR-45 ADPKD-10 RR↑-8 Other-12

The analyzed group of 75 patients with kidney graft functioning over 15 years comprised mostly males (50 patients – 66%), and 25 females. The mean time of functioning graft in the analyzed group of patients was 17.8 ± 5.51 years. 45 (60%) patients had compatibility of sex between recipient and donor.

The sex-incompatible group comprised mostly male donors (21 cases) and only in 9 of these cases there was a female donor. This observation can be supported by data available elsewhere in literature stating that in such cases female kidneys are less "valuable". The mean age of the recipient and donor was similar and it was appropriately: recipient 34 years (SD ± 11.58) and donor – 37 years (SD ± 11.76). Cold ischemia time (CIT) ranged from 3 to 45 hours (average 19.6 h, SD ± 5.51). Almost all grafts were conserved with UW solution after explanation. Diuresis occurred immediately in 67 patients (that is almost 90%), and in 7-10 days in the rest of the recipients. This can support the thesis that prolonged ATN can influence long-term survival of the graft. Compatibility in HLA antigens between the recipient and donor (according to the A-2, B-5, DR-10 scoring system) was 16.9 on the average (incompatibility: 15.1 points, 2.83 antigens). This can also support significant influence of the HLA antigen system on long-term survival of the graft. Most (54) patients had a level of anti-lymphocyte antibodies (PRA) at zero or 3% before the transplantation, and only in 13 cases it was moderately increased (7-20%), in eight patients it was over 20%, including a level of 90% in one recipient, who then was treated also with plasmapheresis.

Analysis of main diseases in recipients revealed that in 45 cases (60%) the reason for renal failure was primary glomerulopathy, in 10 cases – polycystic kidney disease, in 8 cases – hypertensive nephropathy, in 7 cases – pyelonephritis, and in the rest of the patients it was lupus nephropathy (3 cases) and diabetes (2 cases)

This presented data seems to be interesting, especially because early transplants were performed in conditions far different than today. We treat them as a stimulus to discussion between different centers. As an example we present two summarized case reports of our patients, where final success was possible due to a multidisciplinary cooperation.

Case 1. Patient S.A., born in 1955, initially presented with a several-year history of chronic glomerulonephritis (without confirmation by biopsy). Because of progression of renal failure, he was treated with hemodialysis since 1986. In the following year he received a kidney graft form a dead donor. It came from a 32-year old male who died of intracranial hemorrhage. There was an antigen incompatibility in one A antigen and one B antigen. CIT was 16 hours and PRA of the recipient was 0%. Diuresis occurred immediately after transplantation and biochemical parameters quickly normalized and remain normal until today despite a not-intensive immunosuppressive regimen (CyA, steroids, periodically additional azathioprine). In the post-transplantation period the patient was diagnosed with: duodenal ulcer with active Helicobacter pylori infection and recurrent bleeding from ulcer, two septic episodes, multinodular goiter with thyrotoxicosis, HCV infection, type 2 diabetes, giardiasis, infective endocarditis with subsequent involvement of aortic valve requiring cardiac surgery, and multiple myeloma complicated by a compressive vertebral fracture. Despite these problems the patient has been in a stable clinical condition for the last several years. His hematologic and cardiologic status is stable and he has an excellent function of the kidney graft with creatinine level at 1,2 mg% and eGFR at 75 ml/min. Thanks to periodic cytostatic treatment with Alkeran a significant multi-year remission of the neoplastic process was achieved. This favorable outcome of the disease, despite multiple clinical problems, was possible due to a multidisciplinary approach and excellent cooperation with the patient and his positive mental status (the patient is a 'born optimist').

Case 2. Patient S.K., with a diagnosis of chronic glomerulonephritis (without confirmation by biopsy) with subsequent chronic renal failure. Because of disease progression he started chronic hemodialysis in 1990. During this treatment patient had two episodes of cholangitis. In April 1992, a cadaveric kidney transplant was performed. The donor was a 44-year-old male who died of stroke. Antigen incompatibility involved one A antigen and two B antigens. CIT was 24 hours and PRA of the recipient was 0%. He was treated initially with CyA, steroids and azathioprine, which was substituted with a reduced dose of mycophenolate mofetil (1g / day) in the recent years. Diuresis occurred immediately after the transplantation and dialysis was not necessary. Cholecystectomy was performed in 2001 because of cholecystolithiasis and cholangitis.

One year later a surgical revision and removal of a gallstone from a bile duct was necessary due to recurrence of cholelithiasis with inflammation. In 2004 a resection of almost half of liver was performed with subsequent use of Kehr's drainage for many weeks because of abscesses and continued cholangitis. The patient also received several weeks of targeted antibiotic therapy. Currently the condition of the patient is good, he has no complaints, he goes to work, there is a good function of liver (with no inflammation) and a fairly good function of kidney graft (creatinine 2,2 mg%, GFR 33 ml/min). Conservative immunosuppressive treatment is continued (CyA, steroids).

DISCUSSION

It seems that our good results come from a combination of several factors.

First of all, a multidisciplinary approach to our patients should be emphasized. This approach is a cooperation in a team of nurses and physicians of different specialties (anesthesiologists, surgeons, nephrologists, immunologists) as well as lab personnel. In our center there is also a principle that a particular patient is managed and followed by the same physician – often before kidney failure occurs, after it does occur, during hemodialysis and after kidney transplantation – which undoubtedly has a positive influence on final effect of treatment. Such management not only enables optimal treatment but also favors a good relationship between a patient and his physician.

Appropriate modern and thorough diagnostics is also very important. As far as possible it can be performed also on an outpatient basis and it comprises typical laboratory, bacteriologic, virology examinations as well as imaging tests such as ultrasound with Doppler, X-ray, CT and MR exams. Kidney biopsies are also performed when required with a pathologic examination using light, immunofluorescent or electron microscope. In our center we have also developed our own diagnostic method of evaluation of external tension (tonus) of kidney graft in order to objectively evaluate its status. This method is especially useful in early differentiation of post-transplant ATN and acute graft rejection.

We also believe that it is crucial to maximally shorten the time of cold and warm ischemia time, especially CIT. Its prolongation over 18 hours has a detrimental effect on the transplanted kidney and significantly increases the risk of ATN and graft rejection. This remains consistent with literature data. One of our co-workers, in her article, has compared significance of length of CIT and better HLA matching between the donor and the recipient. She concluded that maximal shortening of cold ischemia time is significantly more important than optimal HLA matching.

Anyway, we appreciate the value of optimal immunologic matching, (especially in the terms of DR antigens), level of recipient's sensitiveness (PRA, subsequent transplantation), as well as factors such as: main disease of the recipient, status of the graft before the transplantation, age difference between the recipient and the donor, as well as sex compatibility, especially in the case when a female is the potential donor and male is a potential recipient, which can have a negative influence of the future function of the graft.

Modern, balanced and individualized immunosuppressive therapy plays an important role in the management of these patients especially in the early post-transplantation period but also in the later outpatient follow-up. Therapeutic options include: thymoglobulin, ATG and basiliximab in the induction, as well as steroids, mycophenolates, calcineurin inhibitors (CNI), mTOR inhibitors and recently more often used co-stimulation inhibitor belatacept.

Clinical experience of the transplantation center in individualization of therapy and use of optimal immunosuppressive regimens appears to be extremely important. During the induction treatment we routinely monitor levels of CD3 lymphocytes. Early recognition of developing infections (CMV, BK, fungal), adjustment of dose of used steroids (including sometimes the need for their withdrawal), and oncological vigilance are the basis for obtaining a prolonged time of the function of these grafts. One should also emphasize the need for close monitoring of immunosuppressive drug levels: calcineurin inhibitors, mTOR inhibitors or mycophenolic acid (C_0, area under the curve - AUC). Since several years, in our center we monitor the level of mycophenolate mofetil (AUC), if necessary, because we have found that the use of a standard dose recommended by the manufacturer (2g / day) does not always result in an optimal drug level in the blood (AUC: 30-60mg h / L).

Finally, it must be emphasized that currently in order to achieve optimal results of transplantation one must constantly improve theoretical and practical knowledge of the transplantation team and use interdisciplinary approach to patients, and perhaps above all, properly cooperate with treated patients, with emphasis on their commitment and understanding of therapy.

Will it be able to further improve early and distant results of transplantation of kidneys from deceased donors? That is the question. It seems that a major obstacle inhibiting significant improvement in this field is a growing number of our patients dying of other diseases associated with renal failure, especially cardiovascular diseases. For this reason, a high number of kidney grafts is lost due to death of patients with an active transplant. However, this is another issue.

References:

1.Dziewanowski K., Chłodny J., Drozd R.at al.: The case of the kidney transplantation of difficult course – diagnostics and therapy problems. Forum Nefrol. 2011,4,43-46.

2.US Renal Data System. Excerpts from the USRDS 2003 annual reports: atlas of end-stage renal disease in the United States. Am.J.Kidney Dis. 2003.42,4-224.

3.Dziewanowski K.,Drozd R., Krzystolik E.at al.: Measurement of Internal and External Pressure of Transplanted Kidney: An Underestimated Method of Diagnosis for Renal Grafts. Transplant.Proc.2015,47,1692-1696.

4. Lapis J., Dziewanowski K.: Internal manometry of transplant kidney. Wiad.Lek. XL 1987,40,1379-1382.

5.Ramcharn T., Mateas A.J.: Long-tem (20-37 years) follow-up of living kidney donors. Am.J.Transpl. 2002,2,959-964.

6.Chojnowska A., Dziewanowski K.: Porównanie wpływu zgodności HLA między dawcą a biorcą i czasu zimnego niedokrwienia (CIT) na długoletnie przeżycie nerki przeszczepionej. Nefrol.Dial.Pol. 2008,12 (1),17-20.

7.Tarasaki P.I., Ozawa M.: Predicting kidney graft failure by HLA antibodies: a prospective trial. Am.J.Transplant. 2004,4, 438-443.

8.Tekemato S.K., Terasaki P.I., Gjerstson D.W.at al.: Twelve years experience with shipping HLA matched cadaver kidneys for transplantation. N.Engl.J.Med. 2000,343, 1078-1084.

9.Dziewanowski K., Chojnowska A., Bąk L.: Kidney transplantation from living donors: yes or not? Nefrol.Dial Pol. 2003,7,68-70.

10.Dziewanowski K., Ostrowski M., Lapis J. at al. Odległe wyniki przeszczepienia nerek od tego samego dawcy dla biorców różnej płci. Przegl.Lek.1998,(55), supl.1.

11.Dziewanowski K., Drozd R., Krzystolik E.: Monitoring levels of immunosuppressive medications – is it just recommendation or a necessity? Postępy Nauk Medycznych 2014,XXVII (2) 81-84.

12.KDIGO Clinical Practice Guideline for Care of Kidney Transplant Recipients. Am. J.Transplant.2009,9(suppl.3)19-20.

13.Brodziak K., Hrick D.: Minimizing the side effects of immunosuppression in kidney transplant recipients. Transplantation 2003,8,160-165.

14.Danielewicz R.: Aspekty prawne przeszczepiania narządów. Transplantologia kliniczna. TerMedia 2015,22-30.

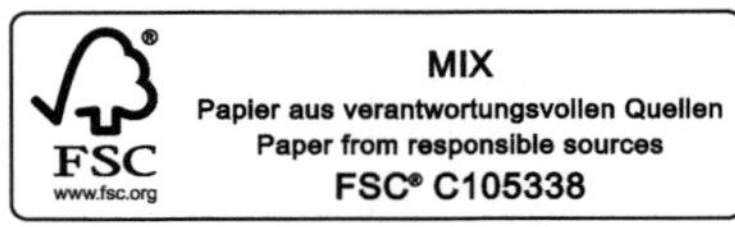

Printed by Books on Demand GmbH, Norderstedt / Germany